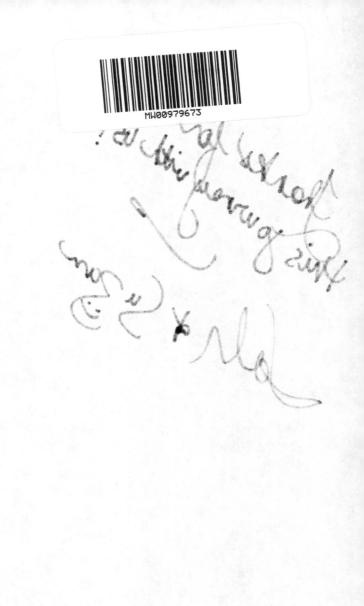

Thanks for taking
this journey with us!

John & Suzann

PARALYZED WITHOUT WARNING

A Couple's Journey Back from Guillain-Barré Syndrome

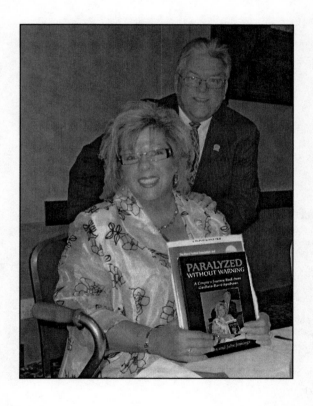

Suzan and John Jennings

Order this book online at www.trafford.com
or email orders@trafford.com

Most Trafford titles are also available at major online book retailers.

Full color e-book version (ISBN: 978-1-4669-6648-2) also available.

Printed in the United States of America.

ISBN: 978-1-4669-6647-5 (sc)
ISBN: 978-1-4669-6646-8 (hc)
ISBN: 978-1-4669-6970-4 (e)

Library of Congress Control Number: 2012921938

Trafford rev. 03/22/2013

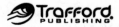 www.trafford.com

North America & international
toll-free: 1 888 232 4444 (USA & Canada)
phone: 250 383 6864 ♦ fax: 812 355 4082

CONTENTS

FOREWORD

One of the joys of my job as a neurologist at the University of British Columbia is the opportunity to work with patients and families like Mrs. and Mr. Jennings. Sharing the journey from diagnosis through recovery with my patients is a great privilege, and not a day goes by where I don't learn something from my patients. The Jennings's honest account of her experience with Guillain-Barré syndrome (GBS) highlights the important emotional impact of an acute medical illness, not just on the individual but on the family. Mrs. Jennings vividly describes one of the most challenging aspects of GBS—the psychological toll of the unexpected, rapid loss of function and dependence on others. Through the acute illness and long rehabilitation phase, Mrs. Jennings has used her wonderful sense of humour, charisma and determination to deal with the challenges that have come her way.

I initially met Mrs. Jennings at the EMG lab at St. Paul's Hospital, where I performed electrophysiological testing on her nerves and muscles that confirmed the diagnosis of Guillain-Barré syndrome (GBS). The tests showed that instead of travelling at the normal speed of more than 40 meters per second in the legs, her nerves were transmitting information at 21 meters per second in some segments. The severe autoimmune attack on her peripheral nerves had caused the acute onset of numbness, altered sensations, pain and weakness. Fortunately, GBS is a treatable illness, and we were able to provide Mrs. Jennings with immunoglobulin therapy, a blood product derived from a pool of thousands of donors, which helps modulate the immune system.

Mrs. Jennings needed a lot of supportive care in the hospital, as well as treatment of her severe neuropathic pain. Without a lot of determination and hard work at the G. F. Strong Rehabilitation Hospital and after, together with her rehab team, I don't think Suzan would have achieved the level of recovery that she did—exceeding my initial expectations.

I was fortunate to experience the minor triumphs along the way—the celebration of the return of a reflex when hitting the tendon with a reflex hammer, the early steps with a walker . . .

Mr. and Mrs. Jennings have been generous in sharing their experience and have co-lectured with me at the University of British Columbia Medical School, where they moved a large group of medical students to tears and laughter with their honest account and received a standing ovation from the class! In her characteristic fashion, Mrs. Jennings has put her hard-earned knowledge about this illness to good use, becoming involved in local advocacy issues such as access for those with disabilities and volunteering with the Guillain-Barré Foundation of Canada, providing support to other newly diagnosed patients.

Dr. Kristine Chapman, MD, FRCPC
Faculty of Medicine, the University of British Columbia, Vancouver, General Hospital, Neuromuscular Diseases Unit, Neurology and EMG

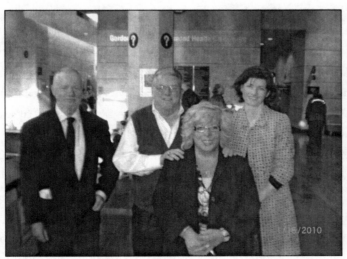

After completing our lecture at the University of British Columbia.
Dr. Chapman right, and Professor MacDonald, left.

PREFACE

When I first thought about writing this book, as I lay in my hospital bed, my vision was not only to write about my journey after contracting Guillain-Barré syndrome in March 2008 but about my life's journey. Although at 49 years old I am young by some standards, I feel like a cat that has used up almost all her nine lives. It was as though my thoughts came to me in 3D because the idea just seemed so "far out there." Me write a book? I'd been paralyzed from the neck down; I was hooked up to an IV pole; had an oxygen mask on; could not make it through the day without copious amounts of morphine and other drugs, could barely speak, could hardly see, could not walk, could not hold a pen, could not use a typewriter—but somehow, I just never gave up and I forged on.

I would like to thank my husband, John, for his patience, kindness and input into our book. He never gave up on me, even when I felt at times I had. The greatest tragedy of all is that we almost did not make it.

To Bill, Judi and Aunt Gerry: thanks for being there for us.

To Susan, Sherry and everyone at the GBS Foundation of Canada—a huge thank you for encouraging John and me to find our voice in helping others.

Of course I would not be where I am today had it not been for the countless medical personnel that worked on me, including Tom and everyone at St. Paul's Hospital, especially Ward 8; the NMS Neuromusculoskeletal program on the 4th floor of G. F. Strong Rehabilitation Centre, including Carol, Marian, Isobel, Nancy, Tom, Barb, Walter and so many more. My medical team: Dr. Chapman, Dr. Finlayson, Dr. Yap, Dr. Badii and Dr. Kostamo. You all helped me find the new me.

A huge thank you to Atlific Hotels and Holiday Inn Vancouver Downtown: Robert C, Philippe, Bob L, Leslie, Suzanne, Arlene, Rachelle, Chef Masa, Tina, Stefanie, Joanne, Bonnie, Angela, Debbie, Maria and many others.

To the team and congregation at Kingsway Foursquare Church, particularly pastor's Barry, Joanne & Dairn, who became our inspirational foundation.

To our friends Janet, Sue, Layla, Lydia, Deb, Lisa, Eleanor, Diane, Anna, Marlene, Wendy, SKAL Vancouver Club, Joe, Andrea: you will just never know what you mean to us.

Carolle, this project probably would have been derailed had it not been for you, so thank you for always just being a click away.

Rick, what can we say but thank you for the friendship, inspiration and support of this project right out of the gate.

A big hug goes out to our dear friends Don and Marilyn. You welcomed me into John's life and treated me as "just one of the high school friends," even though I was young enough to be your daughter! Travelling will never be the same without you and at the time of writing our manuscript, Don was fighting his own battle to live, however, he has since passed. *Mahalo.*

Lastly, to the various family members and friends who reached out to us in our hour of need, thank you is simply not enough, but we thank you. As we have learned, we never, ever know what tomorrow or ever later today will bring, so we thank God that each and every one of you has touched our lives in such a profound way.

CHAPTER 1

Is This How It All Ends?

There we were at St. Paul's Hospital emergency entrance, and all I wanted was my final and dying wish—a last smoke. My husband propped me up against the car as the paramedics yelled at him to move not only me but the car too!

John placed a cigarette between my lips and attempted to manoeuvre the lighter with his thumb over the track, which in theory should have ignited the flame and my smoke. Picture this. I'm propped up against our car, which we've named Maxxi, a smoke hanging out of my mouth. The whole of my left side is completely paralyzed, and my right side is partially paralyzed and is quickly fading into numbness as well. My husband is trying, albeit not too hard I might add, to light my smoke. As a person who had never smoked before, he just could not make it work. There I was slumped over, defeated and absolutely believing I was going in but was never coming back out again. I was going in to die and thought how desperately sad it was that even criminals on death row get their final death wish—but no, not me! This is how the next five months of my life began.

Early on, I had attended Carleton University in Ottawa, Canada, where I am from. My goal was to pursue journalism, just like Oprah. My friends had nicknamed me "the white Oprah" for so long that I thought, *If a chunky black woman can make it, then this "chunky white chick" should be able to make it too!* Funny that my thoughts were focused on Oprah: *How would Oprah handle this? Would Oprah have the grace to fight this disease?*

When I first thought about writing this book, my husband, family and friends thought this could prove to be a cathartic project for me, of course knowing I would have numerous hurdles to jump over first. My mind went immediately to the thought of appearing on Oprah to tell my story—to sit on Oprah's chair. What a dream it would be indeed. Then much to my dismay, Oprah announced she would be returning for only one more season. My heart dropped as I saw my dream fade away.

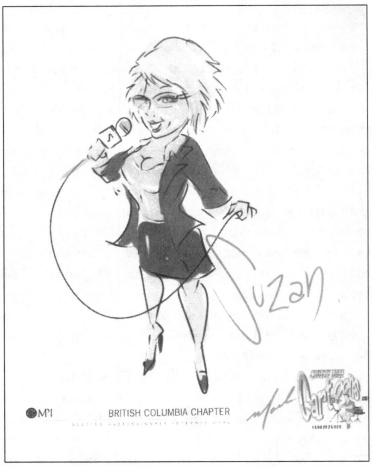

Attending an industry function just before onset of my disease. An artist drew this caricature of me. It just screams "white Oprah," doesn't it?

CHAPTER 2

You Just Never Know

Life was starting to purr along quite nicely, and then 911 happened, and our world changed forever. We just never know what the next day will bring, and I was supposed to be in New York on that fateful day and actually had a meeting scheduled with a client at the World Trade Center for 9:15 a.m. That morning I was sitting in my home office when I started receiving phone calls and e-mails from relatives and friends wondering if I was still alive! I felt so bad because I had not updated every one of my travel schedule changes, so they all thought I was in New York City. Just one week prior, my boss convinced me to cancel this trip because I would be seeing these same clients in a couple of months. We talked about this later, and I thanked him for his intuition, foresight or just thoughtfulness.

A few weeks later, I was approached by my company to transfer from Vancouver to Calgary, Alberta. I originally refused but it was made clear to me that if I did not move, I would not have a job. Due to the slowdown in the global tourism industry, this was not a good time to be unemployed, as many friends had been laid off already, so as a newly separated woman, I accepted the imminent transfer and started accepting the moving process.

Funny how things work out sometimes but at the same time, I started smoking again, after six years of being a non-smoker. My transfer order came through, so I guess it's true what they say about stress. I was moving my life, again, to a whole new city and would be leaving my friends behind—friends who had stood by me when my marriage ended eight months prior, and I'd moved to my new home with my cats Mango and Callie.

It was around this same time that I bumped into John at a travel trade show in Kelowna. We had known each other for many years, as we both worked in the tourism industry and were particpants in the Vancouver Tourism Awards. John was the MC at the monthly awards presentation and the yearly awards breakfast, and I was the representative from the hotel community. We had always been industry colleagues, so between appointments with clients we chatted and proceeded to get caught up on each other's events. We discovered we shared the same news: our marriages had ended earlier that year.

The following month we were at another travel trade show in Vancouver, and we sat comfortably again flirting and chatting between meetings with clients, and when the event was finished, John plucked up the courage to ask me out for dinner.

I informed him that as luck would have it, I was being transferred to Calgary the following week. You see, Calgary is one Canadian Province and a one-hour flight away, so that would prove to be a little challenging. We did arrange to have that dinner date the following month when I would be returning for business. On this particular night, I was working a tradeshow, once again, with my friend Sue. John was to come to my booth to say hello and then we would drive our respective cars to our dinner location. Well, Sue had a good chuckle that night because she said I was acting like a teenager. I kept asking her what time it was, even though I had my own watch on my arm. A few snacks and several glasses of wine followed and eventually what seemed like hours later, John arrived at our booth. Blushing and giggling, we walked around to say hello to our many friends in the industry. I am sure we created quite a buzz that evening, and not just in my head. The dinner went very well; it was entertaining and enjoyable. John even plucked up the courage to kiss me, after opening my car door. We agreed it would be nice to see each other again.

Over the course of the next year, while John courted me long distance, we had to face many of life's hiccups, one of which being our age difference. There are 18 years between us; I was young enough to be his daughter. How we found out about our age gap was during one of our nightly phone calls (we used to talk for at least one hour per night, no matter where we were in the world) when John mentioned he'd graduated from high school in June 1961. That was the year I was born!

I asked, "Well, how old are you then?"

He replied, being his witty self, "You have fingers and toes; you do the math."

When I was almost running of fingers and toes, I gasped! It took me a little while to come to terms with this, and then I realized it was just a number and we had other things to worry about.

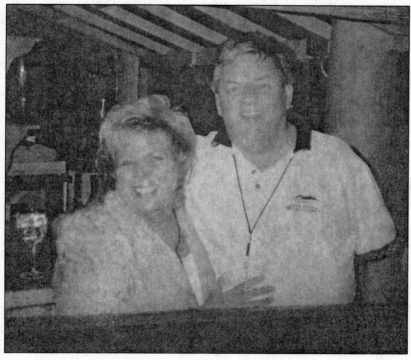

John and I attend an industry function during our early dating days.

Speaking of daughters, he has one and her name is Devon. She was a nine-year-old who was fiercely protective of her mother and father and jealous that a new woman was coming into her dad's life. As I never wanted to have children, I clearly wasn't sure this was a direction I wanted to take. Over the years, we had many good times, but the relationship was strained and wrought with tension.

A few months into our relationship, John came out to visit me for a couple of days. He was so cute and thoughtful because after he drove me to work, he went to the store and purchased so much food that my cupboards and fridge were overflowing. He could not stop shaking his head and failed to understand how anyone could have literally no food in her house—seriously, only ice cubes and a dried-out lemon. With my demanding work travel schedule, I was only home a few days per month, so groceries were not a huge priority and delivery was my friend. As a surprise, John thought he would surprise me with not only a stocked food pantry and fridge but a home-cooked meal. He was the one who got the surprise when he turned on my oven and realized this was where I stored my collection of virtually new plastic storage containers!

A few months later, I suffered my first and only seizure when I collapsed in the coffee shop at work. I was blessed that there were a number of nurses in the cafe who were on break. They tended to me and ensured that I did not choke, swallow my tongue and looked after me until the ambulance arrived.

When I arrived at the hospital, I had "come out of the seizure" but was in distress because I could not see. I was reacting to the light generating from the fluorescent tubes above, causing me painful jabs in my head. The attending doctor informed me I could go home as long as I was not alone. As mentioned earlier, I was single and had just relocated, so I agreed and spent the night alone. I was fine, nervous but fine, and the doctors never found out why this occurred and I have never experienced another episode.

While I was recovering, and since I had to be off from work, John suggested I come to Vancouver for a little R & R and stay with him for a few days. We arranged that I would take the bus from Calgary, and we would meet in the middle and then drive back to Vancouver together. En route we enjoyed some sightseeing and just had some much-needed fun. It was a fantastic break and just what the doctor ordered. It was during this time that John started to steal my heart.

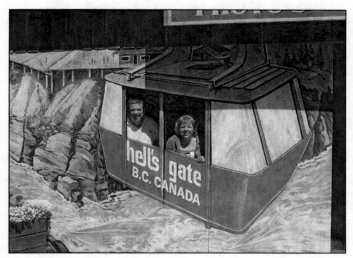

Sightseeing during our R & R trip in British Columbia.

When I flew back to Calgary the following week, I realized my time there was limited. A few months later, during one of our nightly phone calls, John announced that he had fallen in love with me and wanted to move forward with our relationship. I remember thinking, *Well, I have two choices: dig into my heart and allow him in, or run away!*

You guessed it—so later that year I relocated back to Vancouver and started working for another company. John flew to Calgary, and we packed a U-Haul truck, which John drove, and I drove my car with my two cats onboard. We had a lot of fun on the road trip, and I just knew I had made the right decision.

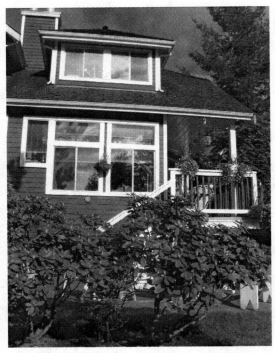

Our first house together in Vancouver.

It became apparent to John, as a Christian, that marriage would have to follow. I wasn't convinced another walk down the aisle was in my future, but once again, John won my heart.

Once relocated back to Vancouver, I started attending John's church, Kingsway Foursquare, and began the long journey of rediscovering my faith. As a child, I was brought up Roman Catholic, but like so many others, what we heard in church was not necessarily what was practiced at home. Eventually I had found other avenues to explore, and God and faith was not one of them. Several months later, I felt ready to explore "the whole God thing" and attended an Alpha Retreat, sponsored by our church. What the Alpha Program offered me was an opportunity to enquire and discuss, in a casual setting and over seven to ten weeks, relevant topics that examined different aspects of the Christian faith. The result of my spiritual journey is that I did indeed find God—or maybe he found me.

Several months later, during a vacation in Key Largo, Florida, John proposed. He did not go down on one knee but was terribly romantic just the same. Everyone—and I mean everyone—who passed us was introduced to my new accessory item, which just happened to be a row of diamonds surrounded by a conch shell.

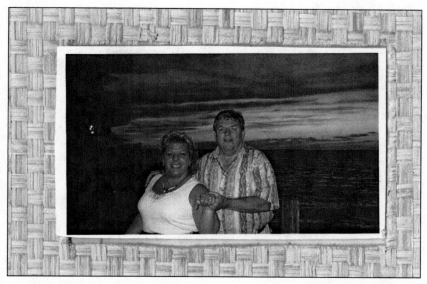

We got engaged in Key Largo, Florida. It was so romantic, being on the ocean, with the sun setting behind us and the table aglow by candlelight.

When we returned, our neighbours were so excited for us they held an engagement party.

John introduced me to many wonderful things, and probably the most comical was camping. I did *not* "do camping" and preferred staying in the comforts of home and hotel—certainly not on the ground, so close to your neighbours that you could tell if they were sleeping, talking or whatever! John, not easily discouraged, suggested we go camping, and we brought his daughter, Devon, and her girlfriend Casey along. They sure had a good laugh when in the morning I pulled out my hairdryer and began looking for a place to plug it in. Our tree was not equipped to handle it!

CHAPTER 3

And Then We Were Married

D ecember 30, 2004, we were married in Vancouver, British Columbia. It was an evening ceremony and had 45 of our closest family and friends join us for our "celebration of our lives."

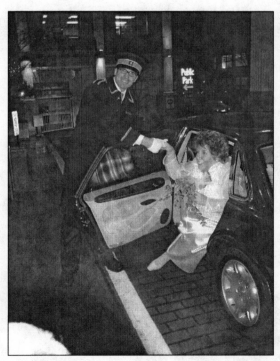

Suzan arriving by limo, of course. The hotel I worked for at the time provided the limo for me to use, plus a gorgeous suite for our wedding night. Thanks Shatha and the Metropolitan Hotel!

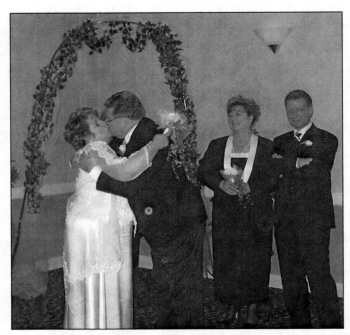

Bob and Leslie, our best man and matron of honour, look on. I was absolutely delighted with my dress because Leslie designed and made it by hand. The skirt was part of my mother's wedding dress from 1948. Mom passed away in 1987, so it was comforting to have her there with me on my special day.

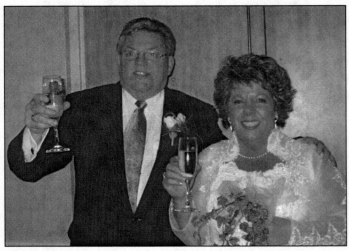

John and Suzan—the newlyweds toasting their new life.

CHAPTER 4

Work and Leisure

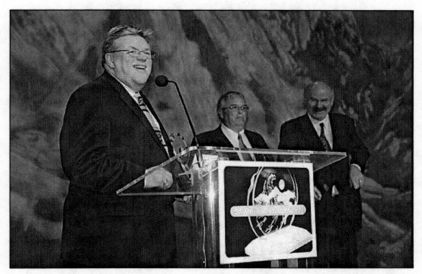

John was awarded the William Van Horne Visionary Award for Tourism Excellence. He shared this prestigious award with former British Columbia Premier Mike Harcourt and Rick Lemon, vice president, tourism, British Columbia.

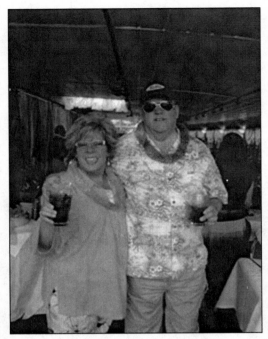

Onboard for a boat cruise with John's work—cheers!

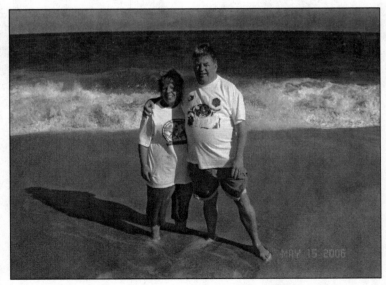

Can you say Maui sun, fun and sand? The waves were so great they lulled us to sleep at night. We both agreed this was the best place in the world and vowed to return again.

CHAPTER 5

A Funny Thing Happened on the Way to Work

March 31, 2008, is a memorable date—it is the day my life changed forever! This is the day I entered the hospital. I had been feeling just fine, fabulous and fortyish; just enjoying life with my husband and our dog Kiki. Then after five attempts before successfully completing a spinal tap, I was diagnosed with Guillain-Barré syndrome. Yes, tough one to pronounce let alone understand. I went from normal to weak, to falling down, to lying paralyzed in a hospital bed in just more than seven days. I *was* scared, in pain and uncertain of my future.

Married only since December 30, 2004, John still introduced me as his bride. That was all soon to change forever.

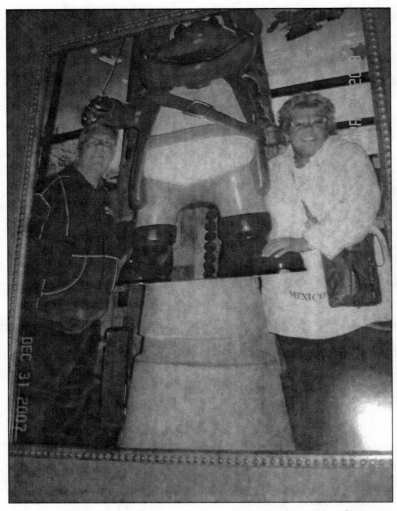

We returned January 3, 2008, from Mexico in great spirits after spending Christmas, our anniversary and New Year's Eve away.

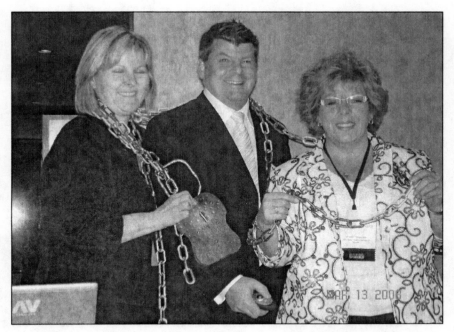

Here I am co-hosting an industry AGM just one week before the onset of my symptoms. I worked in the hospitality and tourism industry for 25 years as a hotel sales executive.

We began to pack, as our moving day, January 18, 2008, was fast approaching. John had started a new position with the same company as a hotel general manager, and we were going to live onsite. The move went painfully slow, and the unpacking part just seemed to take forever.

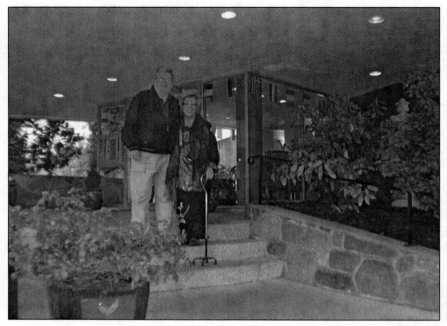

In front of our new home near picturesque Stanley Park, Vancouver (we went back and took a picture here for our book, which is why I have a cane).

Finally the end of unpacking seemed to be drawing near, and we had our good friend Janet over for dinner on Easter Sunday. Throughout our dinner, I remembered thinking that I felt a little off and didn't even feel like drinking my wine, which really was not like me at all! As it turned out, this was the onset of my symptoms, and you can see the left side of my face is just starting to droop. Little did we know the difficult journey that would lie ahead of us.

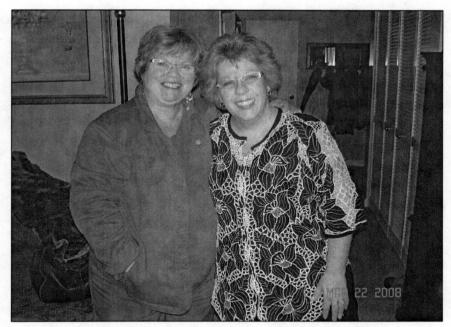

Our dear friend Janet visits us for dinner—the first onset of symptoms.

The next morning I woke with my left cheek tingling and feeling numb, followed by the same feeling in my left arm the day after that. I thought perhaps I was sleeping wrong and that would explain why my face and arm felt this way. I remember telling my husband how weird I was feeling, and he told me it wasn't like me to complain. I remember thinking I was not a complainer but a doer, so I tried not to think about it, and I just continued to "do." But honestly, by the day after that, my left foot now joined the rest of the party. By this time, the whole of my left side was tingling, numb, like when your leg falls asleep and you're just waiting for it to wake up.

Obviously concerned, I called my doctor and explained my symptoms, and he asked me to come straight in. While walking down the stairs to our garage, I noticed my left foot was dragging and seemed to have a mind of its own. Then when I opened my car door and proceeded to sit and swing my legs into the car, my left foot was once again doing its own thing and required a manual assist to lift my leg.

It felt like it took me forever to walk to his office, like I was carrying lead weights. My doctor came in and proceeded to tap my elbows and ankles, gave me a cursory look over and told me I was working too hard and that I was fine and to just go home and relax!

I told him this did not make sense, as I was feeling lethargic, had absolutely no energy, my left side felt hard as a rock, I had virtually no feeling in the left side and I couldn't even hold a tea cup or a pen in my left hand.

Without missing a beat, he said, "You're right handed? Use your right hand and just relax."

I told him I had an appointment with my chiropractor and massage therapist in two days, and he thought this to be a good idea. He told me to stay the course, sent me for blood tests and asked me to call him the next day for the results, which I did. They came back fine.

The next two days were horrendous for me. I tried to concentrate on working, as I worked from a home office. I thought it would help take my mind off what may be wrong with me and instead help me focus on my strengths.

Did I trust my back carrying my heavy briefcase? Stress is an easy answer. I tried a heating pad, ice pack, sitting, standing; lying down . . . . there was just no position remotely comfortable. Still I forged on.

One of my passions is what's called "cold calling" in the sales profession. Nothing thrilled me more than picking up the phone to start the long sales cycle of finding out who may be doing business in your area, narrowing down who your correct contact may be and then actually calling him or her. For most sales professionals this is a truly terrifying part because you could be shut down at any point during this process by not engaging your prospective client right from the start. So off I went. I took a "lead sheet" and started this process. The problem was, it pretty much required two hands, and I only had my right hand working. This proved to be challenging, but I forged ahead and actually made quite a few calls over those last few days. Inside I was scared, but outwardly I was stoic and simply made the decision to try. Just try. In the end, that is all we can ever really do, right?

CHAPTER 6

I Take the Fall That Started It All

The next two days I continued to drive and work, even though it was becoming increasingly difficult. Just walking up and down the 14 steps to the parkade in our building was now a huge obstacle.

On the Friday, as I went to the medical building, I fell at the curb in front of the entrance. It was just awful! As luck would have it, it was a snowy, freaky Friday in Vancouver. I fell face first into a huge puddle. As I was falling, I was thinking, *Oh, God? Are you there? Is this really happening? Why is this happening? Oh crap, I can't stop!*

It was like my internal brakes had just stopped working that day, Friday, March 28, 2008.

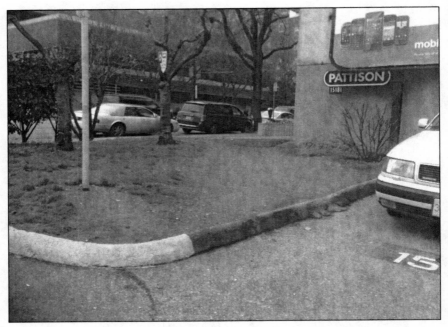

This is the curb I could not manoeuvre over. I knew I had to lift my foot up over it, but my body had other ideas—like not lifting at all. What a mess; I was between my tears and the mud!

Luckily, this nice man came over to help me up. He asked what happened and I said my foot missed the curb, but in actuality, my foot did not feel the curb, which is why I missed it. I was losing the feeling in the bottom of my left foot. It was so weird, because although I knew I had just fallen, I could not explain what my body was feeling or not feeling. The man helped me to my feet. If any of you have ever tried to stand or walk when your feet were asleep, this was what I was attempting to do with great effort, but not with great response. I told him I was just going to wait a few minutes to get my bearings, which I did before I walked into the building.

By the time I arrived at the floor for my appointments, I was a sad case for sure. I was dripping wet from the snow and mud, and I was sobbing. Both my massage therapist and chiropractor looked at me and did not know what to say or do. They tried to calm me down and then thought a little massage and therapy might help. After seeing them, they mentioned my left side was very tight, unusually hard, and said I should see my doctor on Monday. They were as concerned as I was.

I remember walking back to my car, and sitting there all cute and pretty was our dog Kiki. I was thinking, *this could be the last time I drive my car with you*—and, in fact, March 28 was the last time I drove my car.

When I was finished with my medical appointments, I drove home and called my husband to tell him about falling and that I couldn't walk up the stairs to our apartment by myself. John even had to help me park my car because it was difficult just manoeuvring that task, one I had easily performed for the past 35 years. This was now giving new meaning to the term "20-minute workout."

Two days passed, and I quickly got worse. I was now walking like a drunken penguin, and walking on my own was becoming increasingly laboured and difficult. John had to stand behind me and take my arms and hips to navigate me. I did not feel I could muster the energy to move my feet up the stairs.

Two days later, otherwise known as my final weekend, getting in and out bed, sitting, standing and walking became almost impossible on my own. John became an extension of me. You know when something is really wrong when you can't light or hold your own smoke. Early on, I remember thinking, *Am I having a stroke?* My mom had been terribly sick throughout my childhood and had several strokes, so I ruled that out quickly as I didn't look the same, but there was no reason for my sudden lack of mobility.

Saturday we had an appointment with our bank for a personal loan. To this day, I still do not know how I manoeuvred it. I had to walk, with John's assistance, down the hall into the elevator, down the stairs, into the car, into the bank building, sit through this meeting and look interested, try to be alert and act 'normal' even when I could feel my body shutting down, walk out of the building, get back into the car, walk back up the stairs (we stopped outside, and I had what would now be known as my final cigarette), back into the elevator, down the corridor and back into our suite. Once we arrived back inside, I started to pray like I had never prayed before. I felt like an outsider watching my body crumble around me, and there was nothing I could do; I felt helpless.

For the rest of the weekend, we made up a little comfy area on the living room sofa for me because I could not get up into our "sky-high" bed. John's daughter, Devon, was with us for the weekend, so she and John rented a bunch of movies, and that was about it for excitement—except when it was time for me to go to the bathroom. This is when you find out how committed your partner is to your relationship, when he has to help you with toilet duties. I can still remember John saying, "I will help you to the bathroom, but I'm not going to wipe your ass!" My paralysis was spreading faster than we could handle, and I now could not use my arms or hands, so there was no way I could wipe myself. In that instant, my role as bride was to change in my husband's eyes forever, as he was now my caregiver.

Monday morning, March 31, 2008, I called my boss, Jim, to let him know I wasn't feeling any better and, in fact, was worse and that I was waiting for my doctor's office to open. He graciously advised me not to worry and to take my time, but deep down I knew there was something terribly, seriously wrong with me.

Eight forty-five a.m. finally came and I called my doctor and brought him up to date on my body's deterioration. Although it seemed bizarre, very quickly he said, "You do not have time to wait for an ambulance; get John to drive you to St. Paul's emergency immediately, and when you arrive there, tell them you have to see a neurologist *stat*!"

We commenced the greatest and most challenging adventure of our lives. Our immediate ordeal was to get to our car because, you see, no matter which way we wanted to leave our building, there were stairs. John lifted me up from the couch, moved me in front of him and placed his arms under mine, and like an injured football player is taken off the field, he took my arms and hips and navigated me like a rag

24

doll. I was getting weaker very rapidly, so time was of the essence. My body was not bending like Gumby anymore and was instead becoming more like stone by the minute.

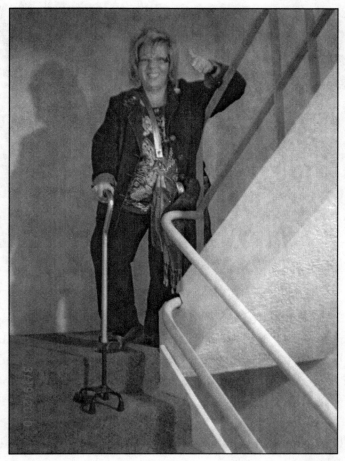

Long after I left the hospital, we went back to say hi to everyone at the hotel and to grab a photo of the exact stairs my darling husband dragged me down.

We arrived at St. Paul's Hospital emergency entrance, and all I wanted was my final and dying wish—a last smoke. My husband propped me up against the car as the paramedics yelled at him to move not only me but the car too!

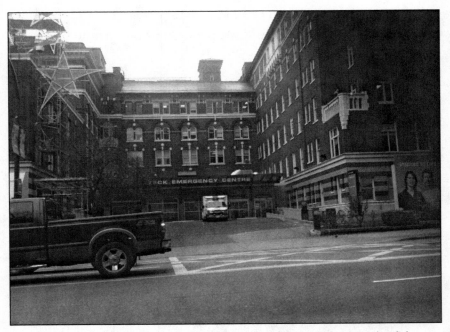

St. Paul's Hospital emergency entrance where John pulled up and attempted to light my cigarette.

There I was, slumped over, defeated and absolutely believing I was going in and never coming back out. By now, not only the ambulance drivers but the security guards were yelling at us. All I wanted to do was yell back at them something snarky, like, "Gee, dude, do you really think I want to be slumped over my car like this? While we're at it, how about supplying a light and that will speed the whole process up, okay?" Unfortunately, my voice was already being affected, and I was barely audible. I was going in to die and I thought how desperately sad it was that even criminals on death row get their final dying wish—but no, not me! This was how the next five months of my life began.

John walked me in like I was a rag doll, although it was more like a shuffle and he sat me down and propped me up on a chair in the waiting area of the emergency room while he parked the car. While sitting there, I was doing my absolute best to not fall over and was probably looking like someone who was terribly inebriated, as opposed to someone who was terribly ill. My thoughts were running away with me faster than I knew my legs could. I started to reflect on my life. What did I have? What was wrong with me? *Is this how my life is going to end?* In a funny-strange (not funny-ha-ha) way, I felt at peace because either way, it was where I needed to be.

Minutes later (although it did seem like an eternity because I was working so hard to stay sitting upright), John came back, and we shuffled over to the triage nurse and began to explain my symptoms and how I was feeling. When we were finished, she asked me if I could walk over to the waiting area, but we suggested she hold one side of me up and John would handle the other side. Well, we didn't get very far when *bam*! Down I went with my legs spread out, lying on the floor resembling a baby foal being born: one leg going one way and the other one in a different direction and unable to get back up. I truly think this saved my life. That is surely one quick way to get attention at a hospital—just collapse right there. I mean, they had no choice but to address my needs or walk over me. I was pleased they opted for option one.

My breathing was affected, and I was scared to death for the first but not the last time. I wished I would just die, because whatever this was, it was scary, and the unknown terrified me.

Within minutes, a gurney was brought over and several people just grabbed me and hoisted me onto it. I felt like I was guest starring in an episode of *House* because groups of doctors would come to see me and ask me all kinds of questions, many of which were repeated over and over during this initial 18-hour period.

Questions like:

"When did you have your first symptom?"

"Seven days ago."

"Have you been outside the country within the last six weeks?"

"No." (Interesting because we had been to Mexico earlier that year.*)*

"Have you had any surgeries lately?"

"No."

"Have you had diarrhoea prior to the onset?"

"No."

And on and on it went. Each doctor would ask the same questions:

"Can you follow my finger with your eyes?"

"No."

"Can you feel this?" (As he tapped my forehead.)

"No, not really."

"Do you feel this prick or this pressure?"(On my feet.)

"No."

"Can you swallow?"

"Not much."

"Can you move your legs?"

"No."

"Can you move your arms?"

"No."

"Do you have any pain?"

"Yes."

I was in a temporary emergency room, and in walked our personal physician, the one who'd sent me home to "relax" five days prior. You have to appreciate the fact that he is a striking six feet four inch doctor, originally from Ireland, and he is standing over me as all this action was taking place. He had tears in his eyes. He apologized to John and me for not recognizing my symptoms and was sorry because I had lost four very important days. You see, in the thirty-two years of his general practice, he had never encountered a patient exhibiting these symptoms. It turns out I had the symptoms of a relatively rare condition that affects only about one person per hundred thousand. John used to always joke around that I was "one in million." Well it turns out I was actually only one in a hundred thousand!

After my doctor left, question period resumed.

"No, I did not have the flu."

"No, I did not have the flu shot."

"No, I did not have any vaccination shots within the last six weeks."

At the time I didn't realize the significance of these questions. GBS can, in some cases, be inadvertently "turned on" by a preceding viral or bacterial illness or possibly an immunization.

While this was going on, I was quickly losing feeling in my extremities. I could hardly lift my hand and was not able to even wiggle my toes. I kept saying to my husband, "What's happening to me?" to which he could not answer. He just kept looking at me with sad, sad watery, loving eyes.

CHAPTER 7

I Hope You Said Good-Bye because He Won't Be Back

There I was. Just lying there in my hospital bed and paralyzed from the neck down. Finally I had been admitted to my room and John had gone home after a gruelling 18 hours in emergency. We had been told they believed I had a very rare disease called Guillain-Barré syndrome (GBS). I said, "I have *what?*" Not surprising, but neither my husband nor I had ever heard of this and were having a hard time even pronouncing it. They told us I would be having many more tests over the next several days.

Imagine if your body rapidly went weak and your legs, arms, breathing, muscles and face were suddenly paralyzed. That's what it's like to have GBS, a rare and seldom-diagnosed neuromuscular disorder of the nerves, which carry vital information back and forth between other regions and the spinal cord. Though rare, GBS is the most common cause of rapidly acquired paralysis and affects 1 person per 100,000.

My breathing was becoming difficult, and every breath felt like a knife plunging into my lungs. My voice was beginning to sound like a mere whisper, and anyone who knows me agrees that my voice is anything but a whisper! My room was dark, except for the light above my head. Pssscccchhh pssscccchhh, the breathing machine purred away, attached to the patient in the bed next to me.

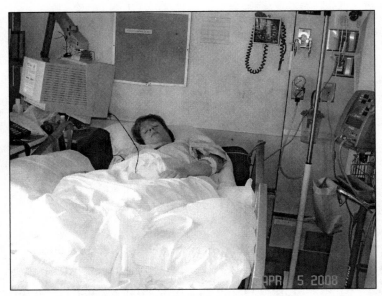

Here I am lying in my bed, paralyzed from the neck down and not even able to wipe away my waterfall of tears.

I was in the hospital. I was unable to move any part of my body from the neck down. I was not able to walk. It has been said that things happen for a reason. I think things happen, and we give them a reason. Roll over and wallow in self pity or face it head on. I chose the latter.

The nurse came to settle me in as best as she could. I concentrated on hearing what she was saying to me. In a whisper of a voice, I had to ask her to repeat it twice because I just could not believe what my ears were hearing. For the third time, she knelt beside my bed and put a hand on my forehead and said, "I hope you said good-bye to your husband because he won't be back!"

I whispered back, "What do you mean?"

She said, "When the husband gets sick, the wife stays and looks after him because it's our nurturing way. When the wife gets sick, the husband cannot deal with it; he leaves and does not come back!"

I was being set up for failure right from the beginning. Not only was I lacking family support, now I was feeling whatever strength I had left being sucked right out of me.

It truthfully took a few minutes for me to digest this piece of information. *Have I really just said good-bye to John for the last time? Will he run away like she said?* I was not ready to say good-bye to him yet. I am very happy to report he did not run away. He stayed and helped me through the very challenging journey ahead.

I did not tell John what the nurse said. It came out only when we were writing this book. He was absolutely shocked and heartbroken that I had dealt with that situation on my own and felt disdain for that nurse. You know, in all honesty, I truly believe she was telling me this not to hurt me but to prepare me for what she thought was the inevitable result.

Through this journey of ours, I found not only did I develop a thick skin to protect myself, but even to this day, I have become fiercely protective of John; in hindsight I can see why? The thought of being alone terrifies me more than when I thought I was dying.

This was the ominous introduction to five of the most challenging months I would ever experience. I didn't know what condition I had, I didn't know if I would survive the night, I couldn't move and now this frightening piece of news from the nurse who was looking after me—what was next?

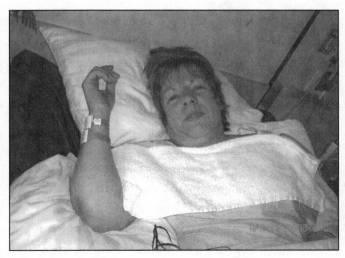

Just trying to be me . . .

Here I was attempting to smile because that is just what I do, and John lifted my arm for the picture. He used to joke that the disease could take away my hands and legs but not my spirit and certainly not my voice; but, you see, I am French Canadian, and I do talk with my hands, so this was a very difficult time for me on so many levels.

Then bad went to worse. While I was awake, they attempted the first spinal tap. Lumbar punctures are always done with local freezing; however, it may not have gotten to the right place! Even though it may not have felt like it, the first needle was Lidocaine, followed by the larger needle to try to withdraw the cerebral spinal fluid. This was the absolute worst time to discover I had curvature of the spine, and because of this, the procedure was unsuccessful.

We learned that to accomplish this procedure, a needle is inserted between two lumbar bones (vertebrae) to remove a sample of CSF (cerebrospinal fluid)—the fluid that surrounds your brain and spinal cord to protect them from injury. The information gathered from a lumbar puncture can help diagnose certain inflammatory conditions of the nervous system, such as multiple sclerosis and Guillain-Barré syndrome.

After three more failed attempts, I refused to have any more of these excruciating procedures unless I was under complete anaesthetic, so they agreed and off I went to radiology for the final spinal tap under fluoroscopy. When the fifth was finally completed, they found elevated protein in my CSF (1.26 grams per litre, while normal is less than 0.45 g/L), and they were able to determine 100 percent that my accurate diagnosis was Guillain-Barré syndrome.

"I have what?" we asked.

John and I assessed my situation—within six fleeting days, I had gone from fine, fit and fortyish to a tingle in my left cheek to being completely paralyzed from the neck down. I was unable to perform the most basic tasks, such as eating, brushing my teeth, taking a shower, getting dressed, brushing my hair, drying my hair, applying makeup, going to the bathroom or turning on the TV. All the things we take for granted.

We would soon find out my own immune system was attacking the insulation (myelin sheath) around my nerves, as well as the axons (nerves) themselves. Because the information could no longer travel smoothly down my nerves from my brain to muscle, I was getting weaker. And because the sensory messages were getting blocked along the way between my skin and brain, I was feeling numb, tingling and in pain!

When I was going through the early days and I was in so much pain, all I truly wanted to do was die. I just couldn't imagine living this way for the rest of my life and said *If there really is a God, then why would he do this to me?*

Also around this time, I had my first EMG (Electromyography is a technique for evaluating and recording the electrical activity produced by skeletal muscles) and NCS (a nerve conduction study is a test commonly used to evaluate the function, especially the ability of electrical conduction, of the motor and sensory nerves) which completed my "prisoner of war" experience because these tests were so painful.

Imagine if your body rapidly went weak and your legs, arms, breathing, muscles and face were suddenly paralyzed. That's what it's like to have Guillain-Barré syndrome (GBS), a rare and seldom-diagnosed inflammatory disorder of the nerves. Though rare, GBS is the most common cause of rapidly acquired paralysis. The disorder came to public attention briefly when it struck a number of people who received the 1976 swine flu vaccine and continues to claim thousands of new victims each year, striking any person, at any age, regardless of gender or ethnic background, making GBS difficult to predict or study.

Although most people recover, the length of the illness is unpredictable and often months of hospital care are required. The majority of patients eventually return to a normal or near normal lifestyle, but some die, many endure a protracted recovery and some remain wheelchair-bound indefinitely.

I was given five treatments over five days of IVIG intravenous immunoglobulin (a plasma protein replacement therapy for immune deficient patients who have decreased or abolished antibody production capabilities). IVIG was administered to maintain adequate antibody levels and to prevent infection. A few days after the final dose of IVIG was administered, there was a flicker of improvement in one finger. We were so excited, and then as fast as I regained the feeling in my finger it was gone, not to return again until four months later—we were heartbroken by this devastating setback.

CHAPTER 8

The "Sharks"

Just imagine what was happening to me. It is as though I was outside my body experiencing this surreal situation. I was feeling weaker and weaker. My voice was but a mere whisper. There were times, like when I took a turn for the worse at the hospital just after completing my fifth day IVIG treatment—all I wanted to do was die. I sobbed when the flicker of movement I got back in my right hand disappeared.

The "sharks" were circling, just waiting for me to succumb. The sharks were technicians from ICU keeping a close watch on my condition. In severe cases of GBS, the nerves that supply the respiratory muscles, the intercostals and diaphragm, are affected, so mechanical ventilator support is needed.

My breath was getting shallower and weaker every minute. Every hour or so the sharks reappeared to check my condition—*am I ready to be carried away by them?* My body was weakening by the minute as my immune system continued to attack my peripheral nervous system, some of which control my breathing function.

Again they appeared. They talked to me about moving me to ICU. I knew I would not give them consent to move me, but as I am a person who uses comic relief at difficult times, I asked, "Can I bring my flowers with me?" They told me no. Someone said flowers would take the oxygen away and someone else said there is the risk of transmitting infection. So I replied, "Well, then, hell no, I won't go!" I truly felt that if I was carried away, it would be the end of me.

Is this silent killer going to devour my body until nothing is left? Would I suffer a slow and agonizing death like I witnessed my mother suffer 20 years before?

It was now day five of this totally debilitating affliction. I lay in my bed unable to move anything but my mouth, unable to speak above a mere whisper, unable to ring my call bell for the nurse, unable to do anything to stave off the sharks. I was at the complete mercy of those who chose to come in and check my condition. True, my husband, John, was there for much of the time, but he was obviously still in shock. He was present, but his expression was vacant and unresponsive.

Like the movie *Jaws*, I felt this presence, and one of the "sharks" arrived and was hovering over my bed. Like all the others in the shark pack, he wore a white lab coat with the letters ICU engraved on the back. I think of many TV show characters who wear white lab coats and have CSI stitched on the back.

It was about this time that John and I had a bedside meeting with the neurological doctor and his team of students. Very much like the TV show *House*, they gathered around me to discuss my situation. As my disease was considered severe, the nerve damage was deemed irreparable. The doctors informed us there was little likelihood I would walk again or have use of my arms.

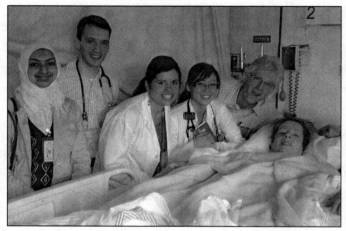

The neurology team discuss my future.

CHAPTER 9

Making a Deal with God

I was not improving fast enough from the IVIG (an expensive blood product containing pooled immunoglobulin from thousands of people—fortunately in Canada it's all covered by our medical system). My breathing was becoming challenged. My medical team had begun the process to transfer me to ICU when all of a sudden I felt the most amazing thing. People talk about seeing the white light at the end of the tunnel. I did not see that, but I did feel like my very being was in the midst of a tug of war.

It was at this time that I made a deal (can you tell I was in sales?) with God and said, "Okay, God, I don't want to go, but I don't want to stay in this limbo world either. Tell you what. If you let me stay on Earth and give me back my will and body, I will devote myself to you and others."

Just at that moment I felt this odd feeling come over me (keep in mind I was paralyzed from the neck down, so I really did not feel much). My eyes sprang open, and there was our dear pastor from our church. Pastor Barry was standing beside me with one hand on me and the other holding the Bible. I firmly believe I would not have made it though had I not found God along my travels.

CHAPTER 10

The Flying Beaver

"Ok, are we all ready?" This was Don, one of the best orderlies in Ward 8, my ward in St. Paul's Hospital. He and my other nurse were installing me into the lift in order to transfer me from my bed to the wheelchair. Being totally paralyzed, I could not contribute anything to the process except to give verbal encouragement (with a few unwanted suggestions on how to do it properly).

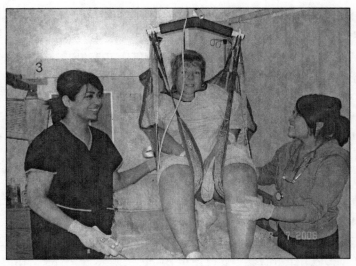

I am flying through the air with the greatest of ease . . . all joking aside; this is an extremely crude way of moving patients who are paralyzed. Its bad enough you are paralyzed and can't assist with the lift, but then they leave all your private parts exposed to the general public or just anyone walking by my door. Very demeaning.

This process was especially frightening since during a previous transfer, two nurses had used the wrong sling. The lift started, I was being lifted from my bed and realized I was about to slip through the sling and fall to the floor. Of course, I couldn't wave my arms—after all I was totally paralyzed. I shouted (as much as I was able with my reduced breath strength), "Stop! Stop! I'm going to fall through!" Fortunately, they finally heard me and did stop and placed me back on the bed.

Nurse 1: "Aren't we supposed to use the green one?"

Nurse 2: "No, we should be using the blue one for this patient."

Oops indeed. The sling was changed to the correct colour (size) and the transfer was made safely.

Of course if I had fallen, it could have been disastrous. Another patient friend of mine slipped through the sling, fell to the floor and is now paralyzed for possibly the rest of her life as a result of this type of error.

The whole sling transfer can be one of the most humiliating processes in the hospital. In a hospital situation like mine, dignity is checked at the door: bathroom procedures in a bedpan that has to be placed and removed for me with accompanying smells wafting through the curtains to all my neighbouring patients as well as many other non-privacy issues.

Going back to the transfer, picture this: I am wearing a hospital gown that does up at the back. I have no underwear on, and then I am raised and hanging in the air for all to see, as often as not, my door is left open. Anyone coming along the hall who cares to look in gets a front row view of all my private parts as I sway around the air, halfway to the ceiling. I would beg the nurses to take my limp hands and at least place them under my belly as low as possible so at least the weight would help my gown stay in place. Trying to make light of this situation, I have termed it "the flying beaver."

CHAPTER 11

My Roommate the Druggie

This one night at St. Paul's Hospital, I was in a quad-4 patient room when the nurse came in to prepare us for the new patient who was arriving: a "whacked out" drug addict who was going to be in the bed beside me! With only a thin curtain separating us, my tolerance level went through the roof! You can well imagine how I took this news, as I was lying there completely paralyzed from the neck down, barely able to breathe or talk, and I was scared to death. I kept thinking, *What if he went crazy and attacked me? How would I defend myself? How would I ring my call bell when I can't even move? How could I scream when I hardly have a voice?*

Much to my admiration, my husband took it upon himself to stay with me for the whole night right on the floor beside my bed. He could not leave me alone, as this whole situation was just breaking his heart too! The nurse was kind and thoughtful and brought John a mattress, sheets and pillows and had him all set up in no time at all with a temporary bed on the floor. John, in his typical manner, made it seem like it was nothing. He made arrangements for a friend of ours to pick up our dog for a sleepover, and then he focused his attention on me. By now, I was looking alarmingly like Linda Blair in *The Exorcist*, except my head wasn't spinning around but I was foaming at the mouth.

My disease had taken over, and I was outside my body looking down at myself. The stress of the situation had triggered a reaction that caused my body to be itchy beyond belief, and I was having constant body spasms. Like being buried alive, I'm alive but can't move. Imagine not being able to move and it feels like spiders and bugs are crawling all over you! I begged John to scratch my scalp as hard as he could, which gave me a respite from the itch, but it shocked John, as my scalp started to bleed. For the next what seemed to be several hours, the nurses attempted to contact the doctor on call to prescribe sedatives for me, and then they actually had the fun job of dealing with me. With enough drugs in me to sink an elephant, finally peace and calm came over me and off to la-la land I went.

In the morning, the patient who started this whole episode was never to be seen again. Apparently, this happens all too often. Drug addicts come in for much-needed medical treatment, and then, sadly, their addiction kicks in and they take off, still hooked up to the IV pole, which apparently they trade for money or drugs. This particular fellow was in his bed area with his girlfriend, and the nurse was asking him if he had any open sores and he said, "Yes, here and there and over here too!" and I just kept thinking, *Dear God how did I end up here?*

As soon as the nurse left them, off they went outside for a smoke and then back they would come. It was actually quite sad, but when you are in the shape I was in, grace is difficult to find. I now know this and am ashamed of my thoughts.

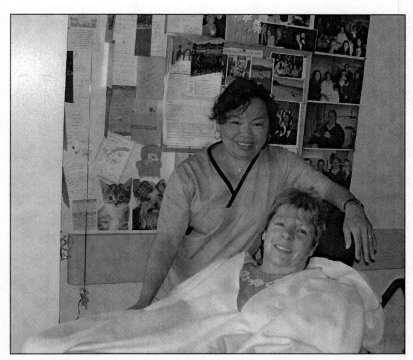

Tom to my rescue: the next morning, when Tom, the head nurse of my ward, arrived and heard about my terrifying night, he came in to tell John and me that from that day forward, I would have 24-hour private nurse care. As he was retiring in a few months, he used the remainder of his budget on me! He will never know what peace this selfless act brought us in our hour of need.

CHAPTER 12

Friends and Family
Make My Day

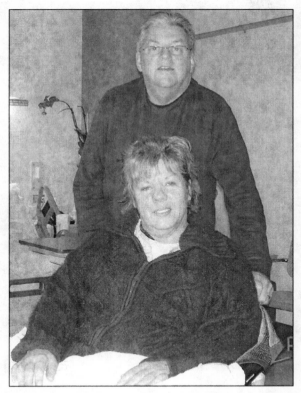

The reality is starting to sink in that this is really happening to us. We're wondering if we will be able to weather the storm. You can see how the left side of my face is drooping and paralyzed.

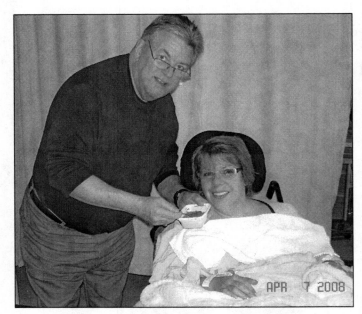

Humbling indeed! Being fed by my husband.

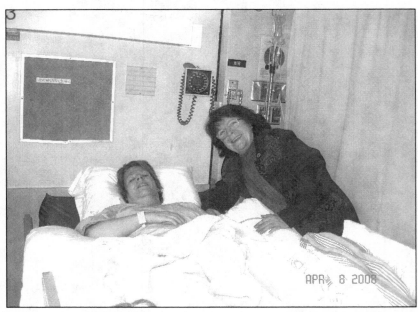

My aunt Gerry came over from Victoria, Vancouver Island, to visit me. She was my mother's sister, and as my own mom passed away in 1987, Aunt Gerry helped fill that void.

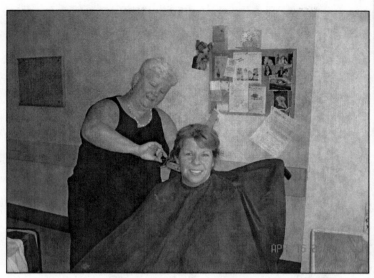

My friend Leslie the hair stylist to the rescue. My "cocktail" of drugs made my scalp so itchy, especially because I was in no position to wash, brush or style it. Leslie came and took care of that for me by giving me a rather pleasant-looking "boy cut"! Coming to visit me was extremely challenging for her, as she had a fear of riding in elevators and, only a few years before, was the matron of honour at our wedding!

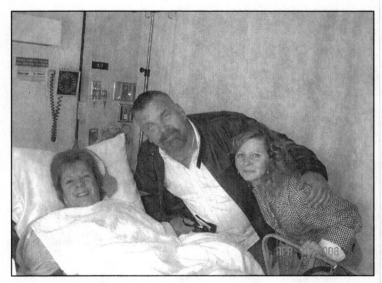

Joe and Crista came to visit and were devastated that I was so sick. Joe was actually supposed to be at our place for dinner that Sunday night with Janet and felt bad he was not there for me.

49

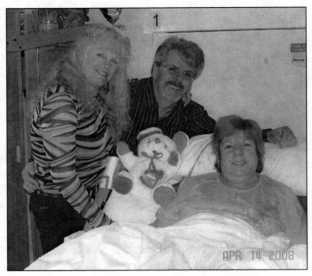

My brother Bill and his partner, Judi, came to visit me in the hospital for the first time. It was so sad looking into his teary eyes, as I am sure he was thinking I reminded him of our own mother, who spent much of her life in the hospital and was paralyzed at times.

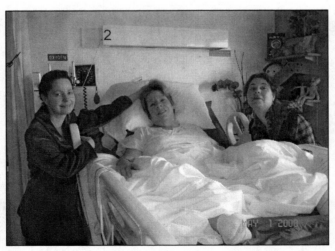

My former sister-in-law Debbie and her sister, Gina, came to visit me. I had not seen Deb for 30 years, since they'd separated, so it was great to see her. A few months ago, I actually visited her in the same hospital, when she was dying from cancer. She has since passed away, but I trust she knew just how much this visit meant to me.

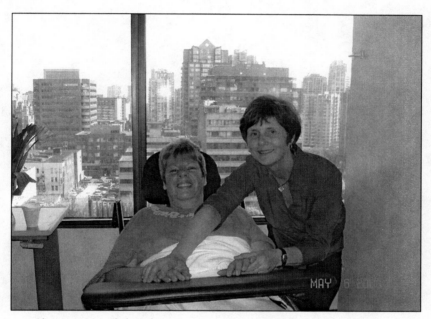

Alison, my original physiotherapist, came to visit and promptly made me work on my posture; seriously—I'm paralyzed, and she's instructing me on how I should sit and how my hands should be for maximum efficiency, and she was really big on me not letting my muscles relax because she honestly believed I would regain use of my limbs. She rocked!

CHAPTER 13

Night Terrors

I was so scared to fall asleep because I was terrified that I wouldn't wake up or if I needed someone, they wouldn't be there for me . . . this left me feeling utterly petrified. I was so sad because I could not wipe away my own tears. Deep terror would enter my soul at night, when it would get dark and all the visitors had left for the day and most of the staff had gone home. I was alone and not able to fend for myself. Left to my own thoughts, all I wanted to do was jump out the window, but I couldn't get out of bed by myself, let alone call for assistance.

I was what they called a "two-person lift"—not because of my size but due to my inability to assist the nurses. During the night there were only two nurses on duty, so when they started their breaks, or if one was tied up with a patient, I would have to wait a very long time, sometimes until the morning. Sometimes I needed a bed pan or more medications; sometimes I just wanted friendly company.

Night terrors would plague me and terrify me. (No wonder, when you look at how some of the nurses reacted around me.)

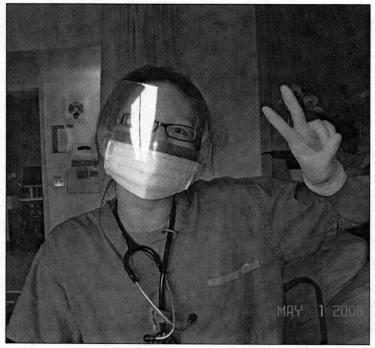

This is just a sample of how one nurse came in to see me because she was concerned I might be contagious. Little wonder why I had night terrors.

I was unable to turn my television on. I was unable to activate the nurse call button for help, and most of the time, I was unable to vocalize loud enough to be heard. I have always had a fear of my door being closed (this goes back to my childhood, and it took me many years of therapy to get over it). I still cannot stand to sleep with my door closed. So can you imagine me, in the hospital with my door closed? I was left with only a mere whisper of a voice, no hands, no roommate—just me and my faith.

Around this time, I was read a quote from Oprah Winfrey that provided great comfort to me "Over the years I've learned that nobody makes it alone. Every one of us gets through tough times because somebody is there, standing in the gap to close it for us".

CHAPTER 14

Keep On Breathing

I entered the hospital March 31 with a breathing capacity of 2.2 and got dangerously low to a 1.1 level. Anything lower than 1.2, they bring you down to ICU to put you on a ventilator because this disease affects your breathing abilities and requires assistance. When this became a possibility for me, I said in my joking but serious way, "Hell no, I won't go." I honestly felt that if it was time for me to go, I was ready and prepared. I had lived a good life, met an amazing man and if this is how my story ends, then that would have been all she wrote!

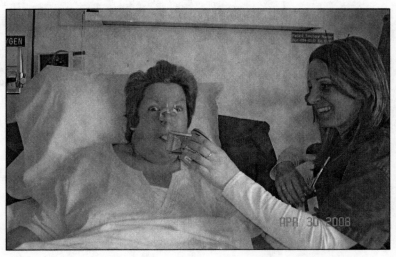

Hey, this is just like a breathalyser, isn't it? Apparently I was not as full of hot air as we had thought! I was trying very hard to expel breath into this machine and it hardly moved. Not good.

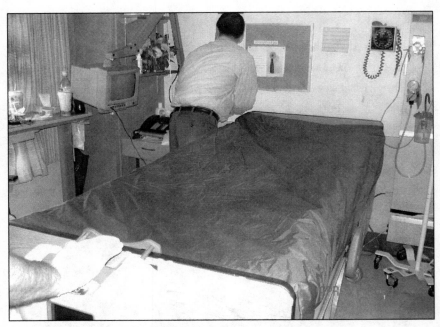

This was my new fabulous airbed, which was amazing because it moved me from side to side, automatically lifting one side of my body up and then the next. I felt like a rotisserie chicken! Another benefit was that it helped with my laboured breathing.

CHAPTER 15

Making Every Moment Count

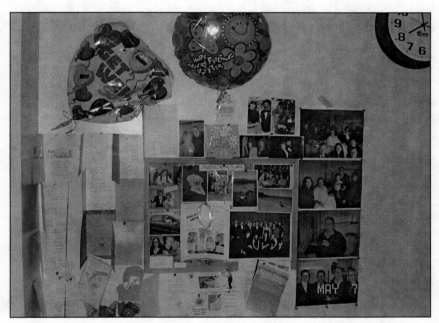

My inspiration board that patients and staff found beneficial. My pastoral team would bring biblical "words of wisdom" and everyone would come to my room after these visits to read and hear what I called "The Word of the Day."

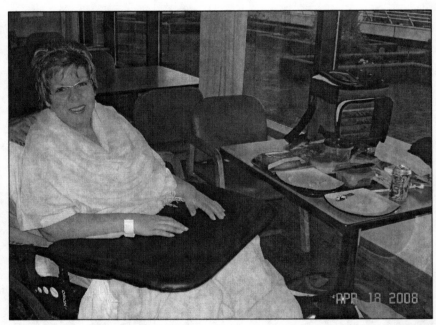

John took me for a lovely picnic at St. Paul's Hospital. John brought everything but the ants and the wine!

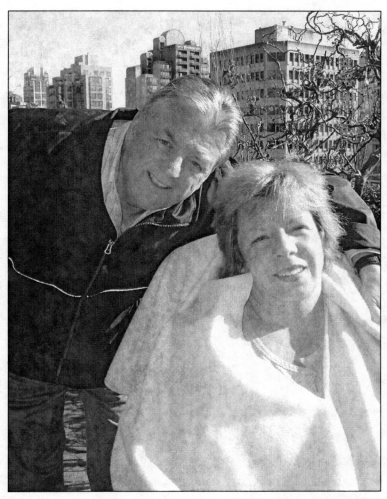

What a treat being taken outside for the first time, and the good news is that I did not even crave a cigarette! (A funny note: when I first arrived to emergency and informed them I was a smoker, daily the nurses would put the "stop smoking patch" on me to help with the cravings, but on day three I said to the nurse, "It's just not necessary any more because even if I wanted to have a smoke, I am paralyzed and hooked up to all these machines; how could I possibly go outside for one?"

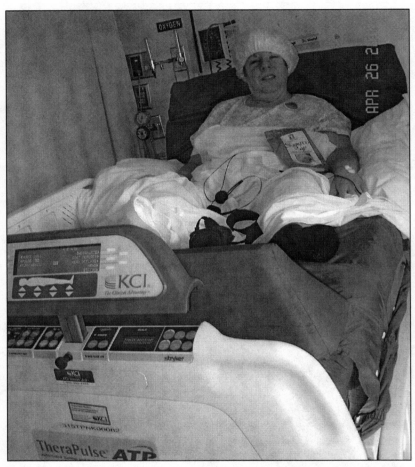

My first shampoo since entering the hospital March 31. What I am wearing is a shampoo cap that actually dry washes your hair. The nurses would put the shower cap in the microwave to warm it up, and then be placed on my head, all the while massaging my scalp. It would stay on for around 15 minutes, removed and hair brushed. It was the closest I came to having clean hair for the first month of hospitalization, and I sure appreciated it.

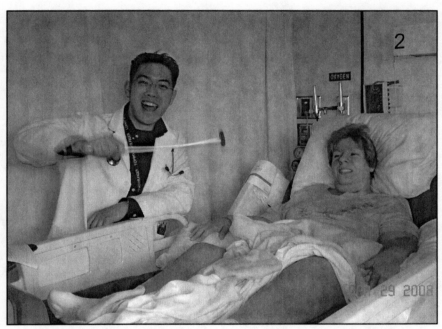

Checking for reflexes again—still not a one! The doctors performed this procedure several times per day.

CHAPTER 16

John's Moment Comes Crashing Down

J ohn and I both lost our parents many years ago. I have only one brother and an aunt who live close by, on Vancouver Island, and the rest of my family live back in Ottawa, so our friends were our "family," our support network. At the time, we both worked for Atlific Hotels, and they were fantastic to us. During weekly Holiday Inn department head meetings, they would add my name to the list of items to cover, such as who was visiting me during the coming week? Who was bringing what to me such as pillows, pillow cases, cookies, pastries and DVDs?

As a company, they took my illness personally. When my husband was awarded the "Sales Team Of The Year" award and was unable to attend the annual Atlific conference in Montreal, they brought the conference to my hospital room. Coincidentally, it was on the same day the physiotherapist sat me up in my bed for the very first time. My head was spinning around and around when I heard numerous heels clicking on the floor. I stretched my head to see who was entering my room, and to my surprise there were 18 management personnel from our company, here, in my room, to present John with the award that he'd missed at the conference. They wanted both of us to be part of John's special moment. For most of them, it was the first time they had seen me since I became ill. After a few minutes, the glass award slipped out of John's hands and fell crashing to the hard floor below and broke into several pieces. For a few moments, there was nothing but a stunned gasp in the air, followed by a huge round of laughter and applause. This was just what the doctor ordered because it provided a moment of relief for everyone.

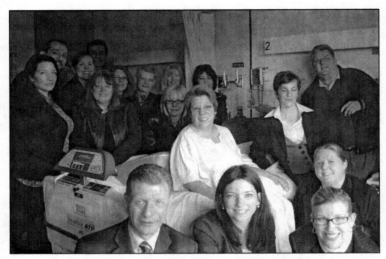

Who knew you could fit so many people in your hospital room at one time?

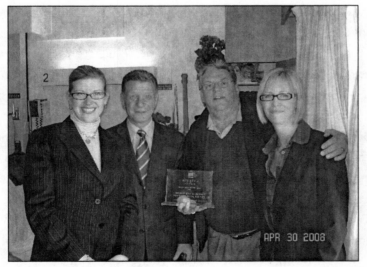

John is standing with Atlific Hotels' Bob, Suzanne and Arlene, holding his award just seconds before he dropped it!

Well, for several days I was treated with kid gloves by all my nurses, and then I found out why. When they saw all the "suits" in my room, they assumed I had complained and these "suits" were from their hospital board. We had a great chuckle over this.

CHAPTER 17

We've Got to Get You out of Here

During this time, I started to experience some small gains of slight movement and some reaction to reflex tests. There was a very small glimmer "at the end of the tunnel." However, I knew there was a long road ahead, and I had no idea if I would ever recover from this paralysis.

I had been examined by a G. F. Strong Rehabilitation Facility assessment physician and advised I was not a good candidate for rehabilitation. Due to the severity of my GBS, I would probably never walk again or have use of my arms. This whole period was extremely challenging; it was difficult to retain my usual positive attitude. Many days I simply "turned on" my happy face to greet others. In many ways, I was "faking it" in the hopes I would "make it." I received visits from the hospital psychologist. The first two visits were part of a suicide watch program that was given to all very seriously affected patients. Of course, I was totally paralysed—how would I commit suicide? By some sort of virtual mind game? When the psychologist made the third visit, she said this one was for her—she needed an energy injection from my smiling attitude!

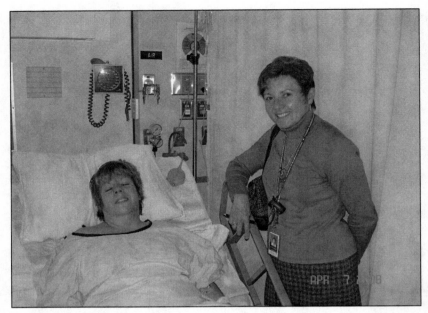

The hospital psychologist visiting me; a lovely person who encouraged me a great deal to feel what I was feeling.

Well, it must have worked, because several weeks later, one of my doctors came in, looked at me and said, "You're just lying there with eyes filled with such hope and eagerness. I'm going to call G. F. Strong Rehabilitation Centre again and ask them to come and re-examine you because I'm afraid that if you don't get out of here soon, you will miss your window of opportunity for rehab to work." Her call worked because within days, I was examined, and the decision was made that I was to be transferred. I was so excited with this renewed feeling of possibility that I sobbed when I had to say good-bye to the home and staff I had known for the last six weeks. There was a great send-off, and John and I were so excited to be moving forward.

CHAPTER 18

Moving to the Rehabilitation Facility

It was bittersweet saying good-bye to my angel Tom. I was leaving the known and moving to the unknown. Change will never occur if we are afraid to try—at least this is what I kept telling myself!

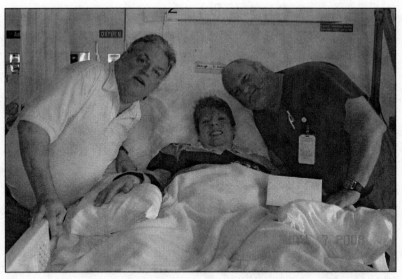

I was so excited to be leaving St. Paul's Hospital and moving to G. F. Strong Rehabilitation Centre. In this picture, Tom the ward supervisor stopped by to say good-bye. He was truly wonderful to me, and I could only hope I would be treated as well on my next stop.

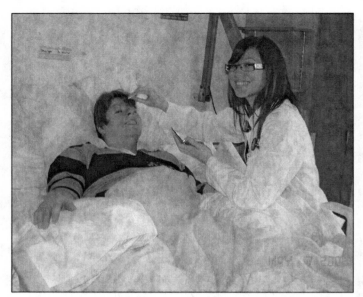

Dr. Angela insisted I get "my face on" before the ambulance came to take me away. Somehow my husband forgot to bring my makeup with him!

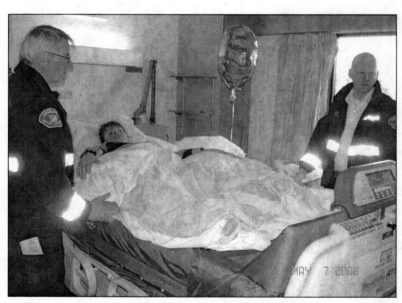

Up, up and away. We have lift-off. Nurses and patients came out of their rooms to hug me and wish me good luck! We were so excited about the next phase of my journey: rehab.

CHAPTER 19

You Cannot Stay Here,
You Must Go Back

I was beyond excited and terrified of this next crucial step. *Would I really be able to regain some of my abilities, such as using my hands, standing on my own, going to the bathroom on my own?*

I arrived at the rehabilitation facility by ambulance, and John followed behind us in our car, Maxxi. The ambulance attendants transferred me to my new airbed, the exact same model I'd previously had, because they thought it would be easier on my body. Apparently, it is very expensive, and the cost not be easily justified. Our balloon was quickly deflated!

After everyone had left the room, the intake nurse turned to John and me and said, "You cannot stay here, you must go back. We are short-staffed. This is not chronic care, this is rehab!" This was like being hit between the eyes with a hammer.

I started to hyperventilate and said to John that I was too tired to fight this fight anymore. I was sick and tired of being sick and tired. I was fed up. I was freaked out. I was frustrated beyond belief. I was so, so terribly sad. I did not want to play this game anymore, and all I wanted to do was jump out the window. What saved me was that I couldn't get out of my bed—I was totally paralyzed!

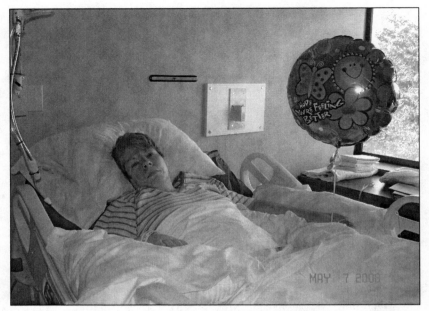

I think this photo says it all! Never in my life did I feel so dejected and unwanted. I did not have a home to go to.

The doctor came into my room soon after, and we explained, between sobs, what the nurse had told us. He gently turned to us and said, "I'm the doctor, and you are exactly where you should and need to be. I'm so sorry this happened to you. I'll speak to that nurse, but don't worry about any of this. You just concentrate on why you're here."

This entire period was probably the unhappiest time of my whole rehabilitation. I cried off and on for many weeks. I sobbed when the visits from my friends became fewer and further between. I sobbed because I felt so alone. I sobbed because of what had happened to me and to my husband. I sobbed when I was told I would miss work for a very long time and would be on long-term disability. I sobbed so hard under the sheer weight of it all. I sobbed because I couldn't even wipe my own tears away.

I was now in the best rehabilitation facility in western Canada and realized fairly quickly that this was going to be the best opportunity for me to regain whatever muscle functions were possible. It was time to (mentally) pull my socks up and get to work. With determination, a positive attitude, faith and God's good grace, I began the long journey back.

That day I had a heart-to-heart chat with God because I could not understand why all this was happening to me. I do believe this nurse was not trying to hurt me, but she was frustrated and obviously felt that having one more patient who took a great deal of attention was far more than she could handle at that particular moment. After the dust settled, I did continue to see this nurse, and she was just fine with me, and it was like the incident never happened.

CHAPTER 20

Now It's Time to
Get to Work

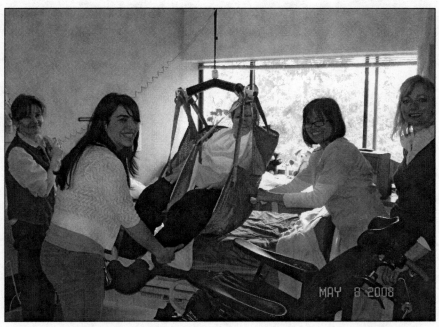

Meeting my new team for the first time. This is how they had to move me because I was still paralyzed and could not assist them.

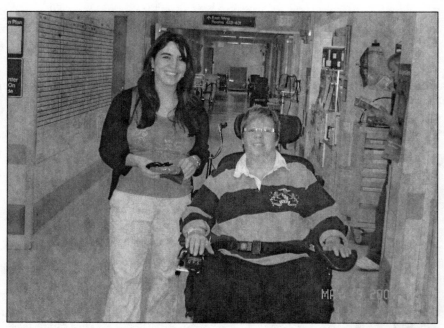

This is my new power chair. I could not move myself around yet, as my hands were still paralyzed, but Nancy is with me to assist.

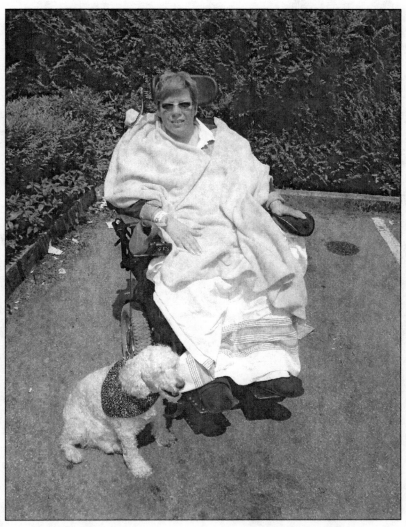

Seeing Kiki, my baby boy, for the first time. He remained terrified of the sound of my power chair and everyone else's too!

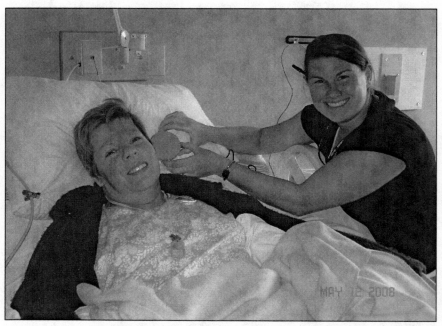

Getting fitted with a TV channel changer that I press with my head/shoulder. In theory this works well except it caused me to develop frozen shoulder and other neck/spine issues, which I am still dealing with today.

CHAPTER 21

Vertical for the First Time
in Three Months

O n this day, my physiotherapist, Marian, came to pick me up
in my room and told me she had a special surprise for me.
I had been around long enough to know this was not going
to be good! She and her team fastened me onto this "tilt table," which
kind of looks like something out of *The Bride of Frankenstein* or *Silence
of the Lambs* (what Hannibal Lector was strapped to). It made me dizzy
but eventually proved to be effective. For the first (and last) time, I was
actually the same height as John!

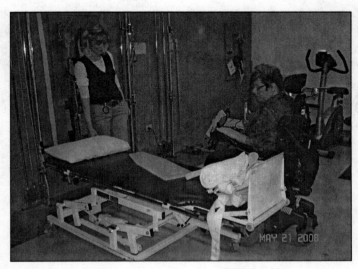

Marian and her assistant getting me ready to go up. Unbelievable!

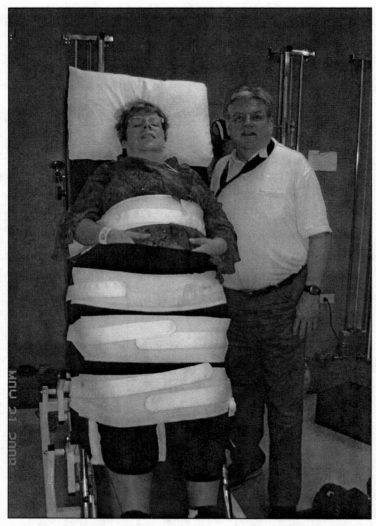

"Standing" with John and looking like the Bride of Frankenstein. And I was as tall as him!

CHAPTER 22

A Day in the Life of Me

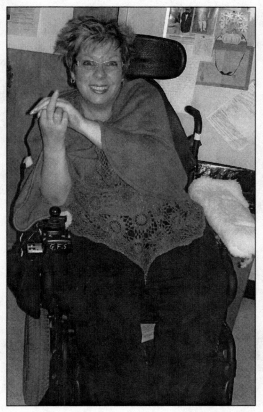

We call this photo "God's great sense of humour indeed." I received the feeling back in my middle finger of my right hand first, and like a child at Christmas wanting to show my prize to everybody and anybody walking by, I would say "look!" and would give them what looked like the "one finger salute."

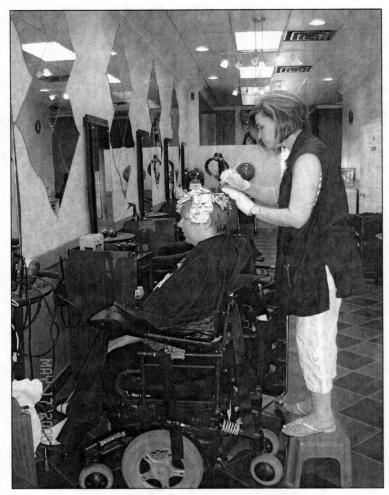

What a thrill. John took me to the nearby salon to have highlights put in my hair and, of course, a wash and cut. I cannot explain how good this felt!

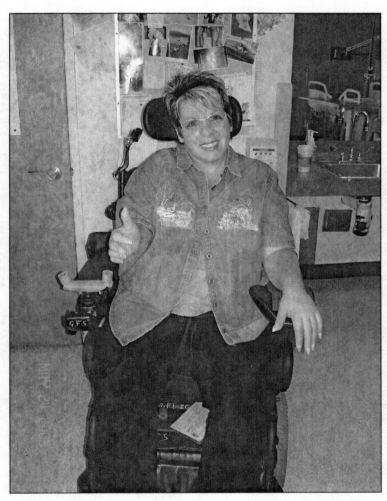

This became my trademark—thumbs up!

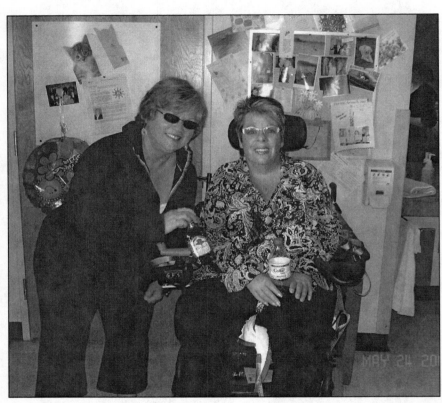

Sista' Janet brought me two of my favourite items: Canadian rye and diet cola. Only one problem and you could tell on my face, I am profoundly upset I can't drink it right then and there! She kept them and, true to her word, brought them over when I was first home. And then I drank it!

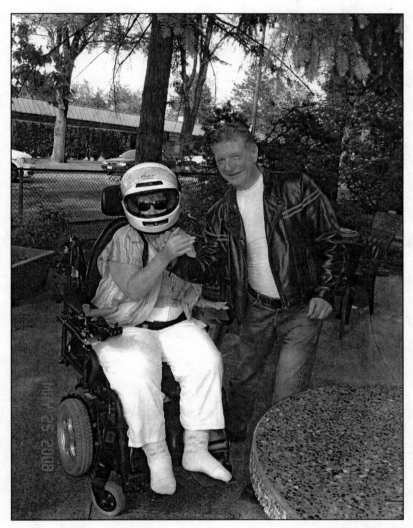

Motorcycle Momma! This is one of my favourite pictures taken with Bob, a dear friend of ours. Not quite the biker-chick look, is it? Little did we know at the time Bob would be facing his own health battle in a few years to come.

CHAPTER 23

Can You Say Pain?

Yet another difficult day for me. This was the most frightening and painful aspect of my recovery that I had to overcome. It scared me so much because I could not feel what they were making my body do, so one minute I am in my wheelchair and the next I am standing! Absolutely amazing!

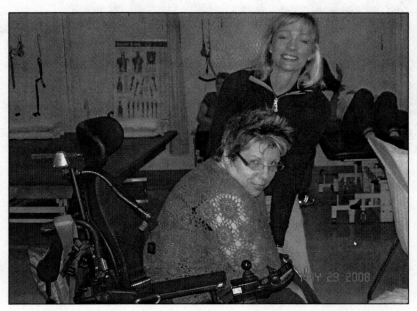

Here I am about to stand, virtually on my own for the first time since I became paralyzed three months earlier, and I remember thinking, and this picture says it all: You must to be joking. You're going to pull me up with this contraption and then I am going to stand on my own legs—the legs I can't feel?

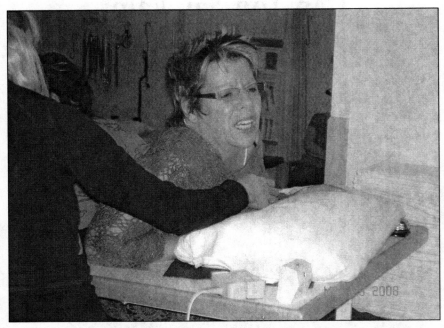

This is my husband's favourite picture of my "road to recovery." He says it shows the whole painful experience in my face, and I guess it does.

"If you don't fall, you are not getting better"

~Michael J. Fox~

CHAPTER 24

A Day of Firsts

W hen they brought me back to my room, after standing for the first time, I was like "bring it on!" I was very anxious and game to try anything. Here I am feeding myself, brushing my own teeth, sipping from my cup by myself. Although it was fun for me, I did feel sorry for the cleaning crew that had to come in and clean up after me. It was a glorious day for me indeed

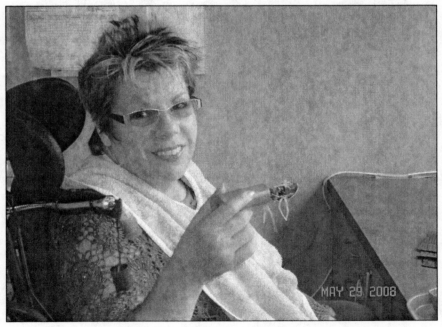

Here I am feeding myself for the first time. More food hit the floor than my mouth, but that was okay with me!

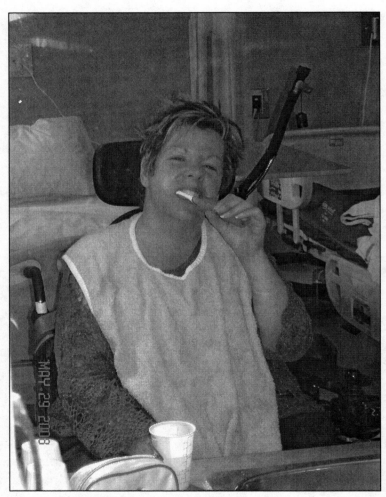

Who knew brushing your teeth could be so much fun?

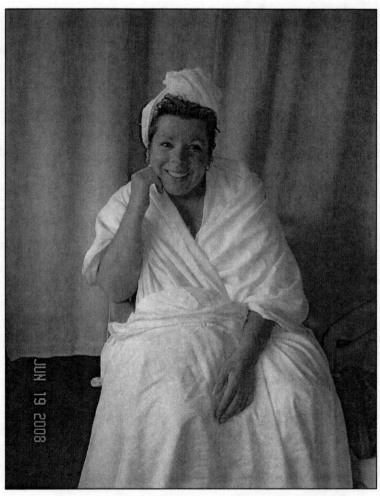

And yet another first for me. My first independent shower. My nurse allowed me to transfer from my wheelchair across the shower bench by myself! What a feeling—I did it!

CHAPTER 25

Attending My First GBS Conference

Isobel, my occupational therapist, brought me the poster for this conference, and I thought, *how can I possibly attend a conference like this when I am still paralyzed?* But I was so hungry to find out more information about this nasty disease that I was determined to go. At the conference, after meeting Sherry and the other liaisons, I made the decision that as soon as I was better and stronger, I too would become a volunteer liaison for the GBS/CIDP (Guillain-Barré Syndrome/ Chronic Inflammatory Demyelinating Polyneuropathy) Foundation of Canada.

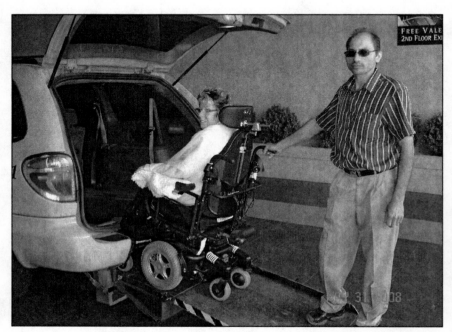

This is how we travelled to the conference with me in the back and John in the back seat. I was very fortunate to have a team that made this happen. Not only did my husband arrive at my rehab facility at 5:00 am but the head nurse brought in two extra nurses to get me up, washed, catheter inserted (which would make it easier for John to handle me on his own), dressed and ready to go by 7:00 am so we would make it to the conference on time.

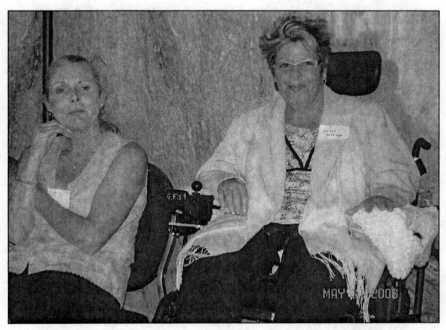

This is Sherry, my liaison, and me at the conference. Funny to note, but John and I attended the GBS Conference the following year in Toronto. Many attendees said, "It's good to see you again." I hardly remembered anyone because I had been so heavily sedated on morphine at the previous conference, but they all remembered me!

When we arrived, I was shocked to find many former patients still in wheelchairs, many still using walkers and canes. Many of the others that were upright, still had crooked fingers, still limbs, halting gaits and droopy eyes. At this time, I just could not imagine that I would recover as much as I have since that day.

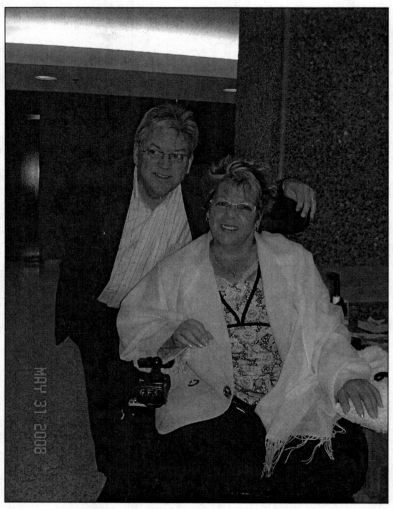

This is one of my favourite photos of us; it just shows the love we have for each other and that we were going to weather this storm!

CHAPTER 26

Freedom at Last

I needed to travel in our car. This would require attempting a car transfer for the first time. My therapy team did not think I was ready to do this, but I was determined. You see, I had been given my discharge date of July 26 and we had to find a home to move to because where we lived, there were stairs and John could not return to his position, as live in Hotel Manager.

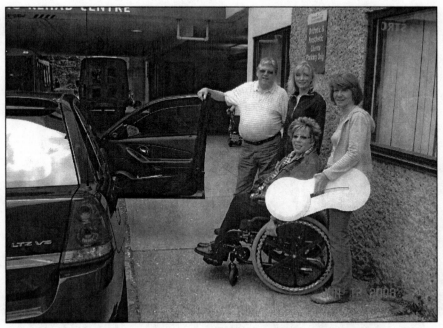

My therapy team get ready for me to transfer to my car for the first time.

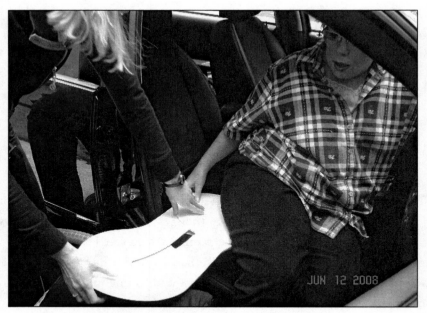

We are at the midway point, and I must admit I was secretly wondering if I was going to end up on the concrete instead of the passenger seat.

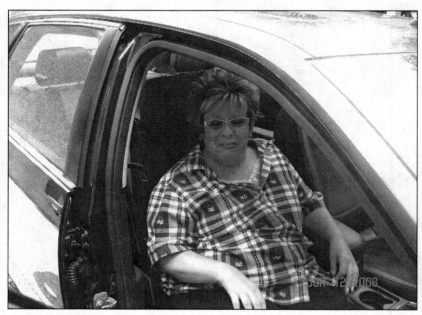

Crying a river of happy tears.

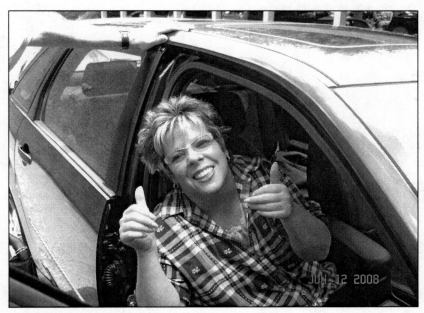

I did it! What an awesome day this was.

CHAPTER 27

Support from Many Directions

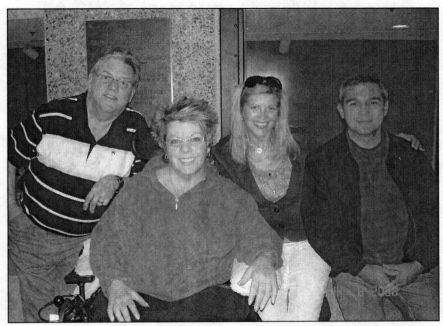

This was a particularly wonderful visit for us because John used to work with Suzanne and I used to work with Kaan. (Suzanne was also responsible for arranging a party in our honour.)

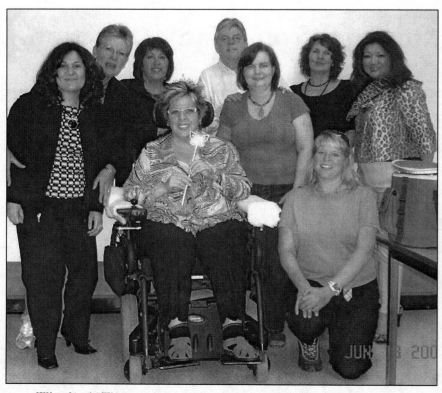

What friends! This was just a hoot when a group of my friends, Sue, Eleanor, Deb, Diane, Wendy, Lisa and Lydia, came to visit me at G. F. Strong Rehabilitation Centre and brought food and wine (a definite no-no). They will never know just how much this meant to me.

Update: We still get together several times per year and John is always our "token man."

CHAPTER 28

Rehabilitation: A Day in the Life of Me

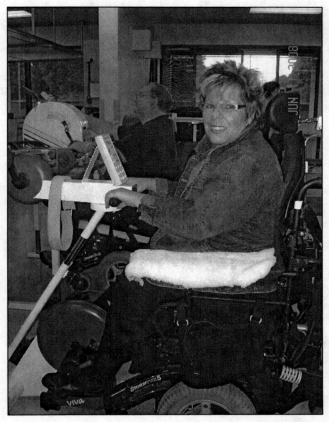

Learning to use my hands—just like the little engine that could, I could!

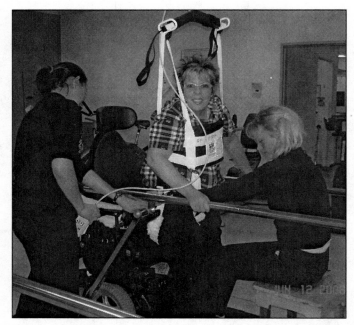

Learning to walk with Marian. This harness would hold me up as Marian, my physiotherapist, moved my legs. Unbelievable. Then the unthinkable: Marian said, "Let's try this time without the harness." I thought she had lost her mind, but the proof is in the pudding!

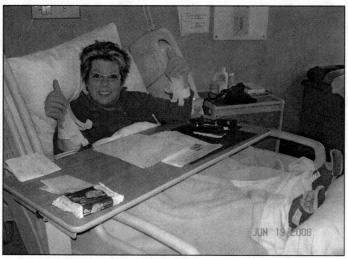

My funky gloves and funky booties. This is what I had to do every day to teach my hands and feet to work again. Painful but necessary.

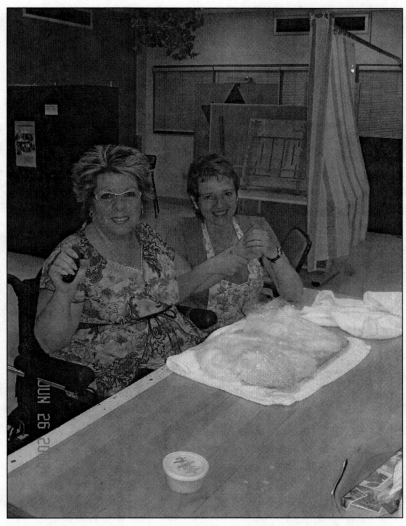

Barb working on my hands and trying to bring them back from paralysis. She would place them in hot wax to stimulate them. It worked wonders because I am able to use my hands today!

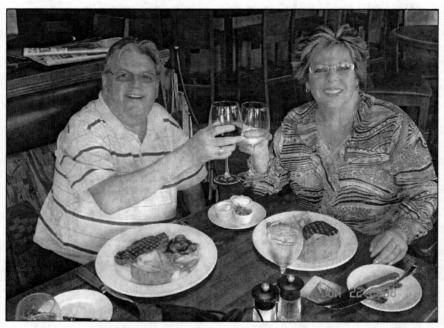

This was such a very special day. My doctor gave me permission to go out for lunch with my husband for the first time, and I had steak and a glass of wine. It was awesome!

CHAPTER 29

It's Party Time

What a party! Holiday Inn Vancouver Downtown hosted a party for us that more than 100 people attended; we were deeply touched and it remains one of the greatest highlights on my road to recovery and in our lives in general. John and I felt absolutely overwhelmed by the love that we received from friends and family. Our dear friend Wendy even gave me a T-shirt that said "Flying Beaver." To this day, when I am feeling blue, all I have to do is think of that shirt and it brings a smile to my face

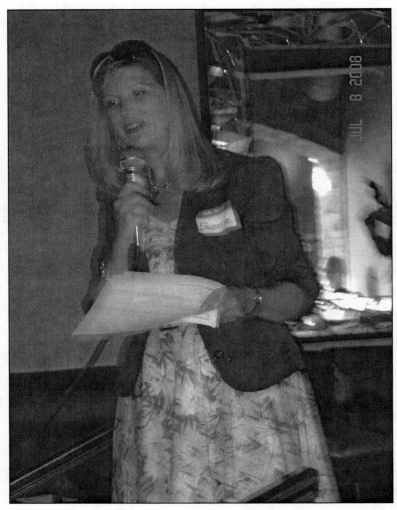

Suzanne, the General Manager, hosted the evening. She was fantastic, and we thank her so much for arranging this party to support us and give us the encouragement to "keep on keeping on."

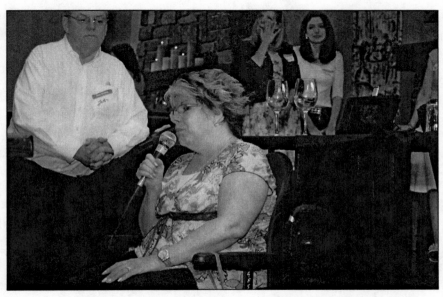

John and I look like deer in the headlights as I thanked everyone. We were deeply overwhelmed. Hmmm, it's true what people say: public speaking is just like riding a bicycle! If you fall off, just get back on!

CHAPTER 30

Living the Dream

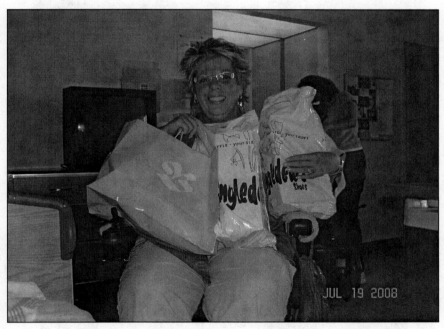

Can you say "retail therapy"? Every girl can relate to this picture. It's my first solo shopping excursion to the local mall. (I think sometimes my husband wishes I had not learned how to sign my name because my credit card works too well now!)

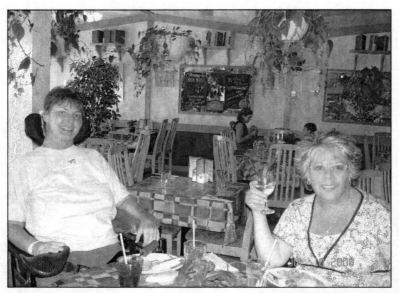

Here I am with Tanis, and we were enjoying our first dinner out together. It was so funny because there was more food on the floor than what actually went into our mouths, but we had a blast!

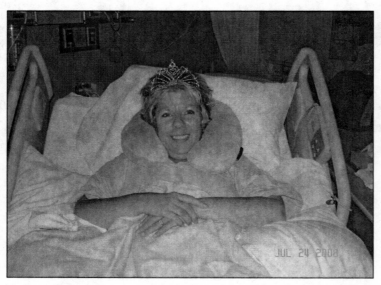

My last night: I was being discharged from G. F. Strong Rehab and this is the princess crown my girlfriends brought me. I really felt like a princess . . . living this most unimaginable life . . . from paralysis and back.

CHAPTER 31

Getting "Sprung"

*M*y last day! How exciting. I was finally going home. But first, Marian had to put me through a series of tests, which I had to pass, including how to fall the right way; this was to ensure I had the ability to be in a "home environment."

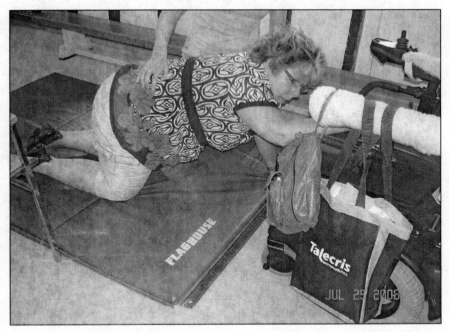

Being it was my last day, Marian had to put me through the paces to ensure if I fell, I could get back up (the odds were good I would fall).

"You rise one day and fall the next. Life is dynamic not static. If I can wake up and say I accomplished something yesterday, that's a good feeling. I'm not special-it's a conscious decision to ignore my pain and focus on the rest. We all have the power to do that".

~Montel Williams~

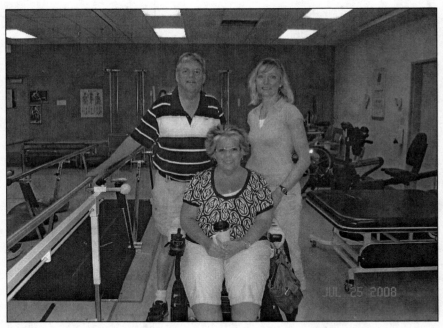

A final picture with Marian. See ya!

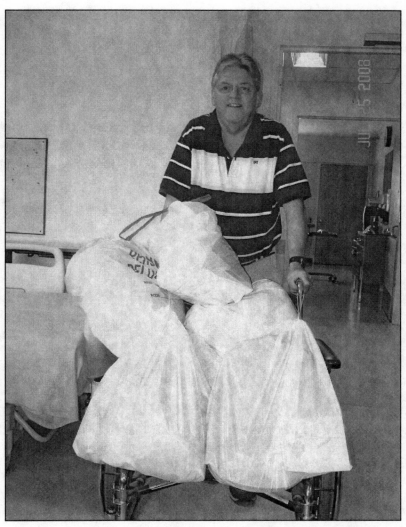

This is one of the funniest photos because I couldn't believe all the "stuff" I had accumulated over the three months—so much that it took John two trips to bring it all out to the car.

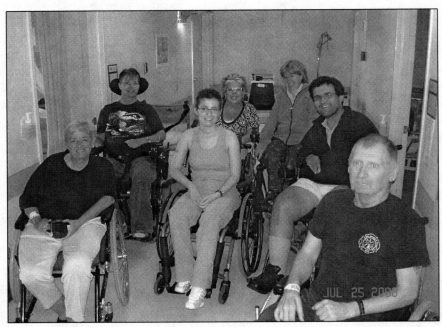

A very happy yet sad moment. All my friends gathered around to say good-bye. It was sad because I was the first to "be sprung," so I had a lot of guilt because I was leaving them all behind.

CHAPTER 32

Coming-Home Day

This was the entry I made about adjusting to my new label, *physically disabled person*:

"It is now July 25, 2008, and I am home. Adjusting from the acute (St. Paul's Hospital) life of paralysis to the rehab (G. F. Strong Rehabilitation Facility) setting. Home to a life, hopefully temporary, of being on disability benefit. Cut off from all the support and visitors I had to a very isolated world with John and Kiki. At times being excited for just being and doing to being frustrated for not being able to go and do! It's like I am stuck between what I was before I got sick to where I am now. Not being able to work—I have worked steadily since junior high school—to relying on John to take me for car rides and trips to Starbucks. It's totally the little things in life that are precious, that mean something. To be in the moment. Just to be here . . . now . . . that is what I must focus on. My abilities, not disabilities. Remembering that God puts these life hiccups in front of us for a reason and that he will only give us what we can handle. Learning these lessons has been paramount as I move forward. Onward I go!"

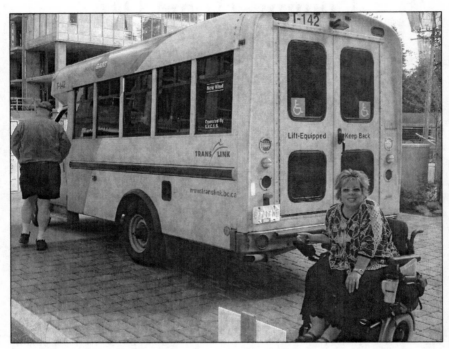

Here I am being transferred by our Handydart system for persons with disabilities and frail seniors. It's just great that we had this form of transport for me because I used it a great deal to regain my lost independence.

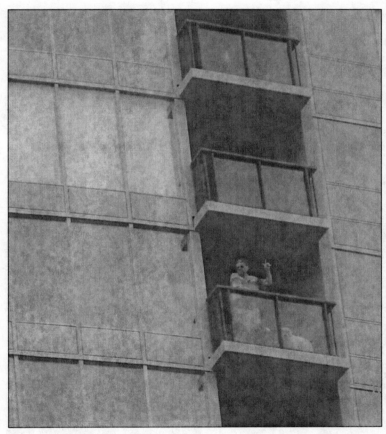

John and Kiki waiting for me on our balcony as I arrived by Handydart.

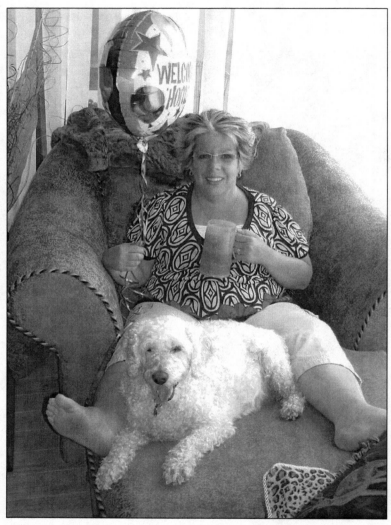

This will always be remembered as one of the happiest days of my life. Coming home to my husband John, dog Kiki, a "welcome home" balloon and a special beverage!

CHAPTER 33

Dancing with My Baby

We attended our friends Kris and Tina's wedding where John was the MC (there was concern whether one or both of us would even be able to attend, let alone John being the MC!). I was determined to dance a fast one on my own and a slow dance with John. The next morning I couldn't figure out where I had gotten all these bruises on my arms and around my ribs and then we remembered—it was from John holding onto me so tight, to stop me from falling, the night before!

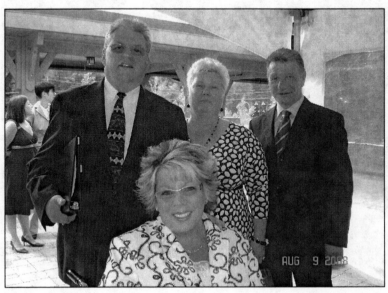

Here we are at Kris and Tina's wedding with Bob and Leslie, who had been our best man and matron of honour.

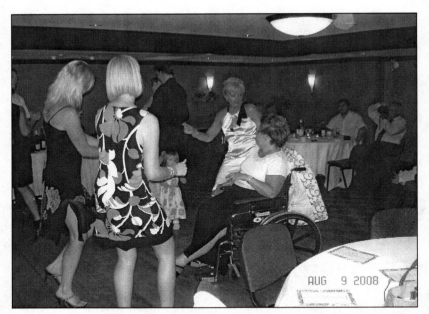

Just because I was in a chair did not mean I could not dance! Rock on.

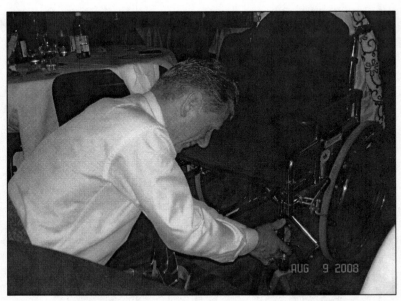

Well, I guess maybe I danced a little too hard and broke one of my leg rests. Bob to the rescue!

122

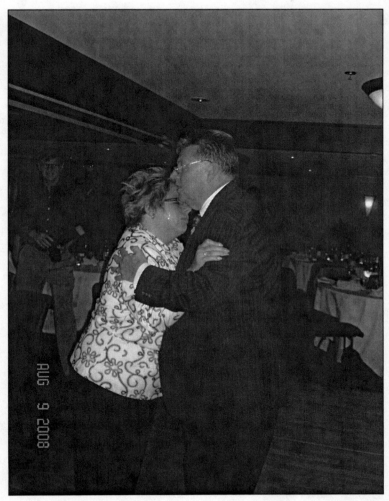

At this particular moment, I did not have a care in the world; I was on my feet dancing with my love, my partner, my friend. I think my tear says it all!

CHAPTER 34

Outpatient Rehabilitation

When I was discharged from G. F. Strong, I attended outpatient rehab at Eagle Ridge Hospital. This was followed by an intense recovery program of physiotherapy, occupational therapy, massage therapy, chiropractor, acupuncture, water therapy and an at-home exercise regime. All of which I continue to this day.

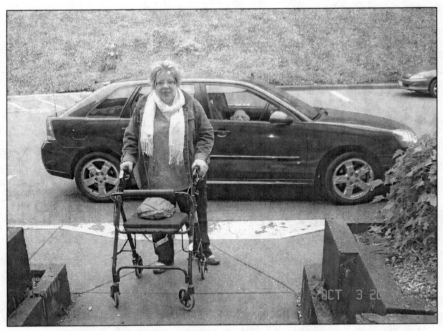

Walking into outpatient therapy for the first time. Behind me in the passenger seat, Kiki is watching Mommy walking away.

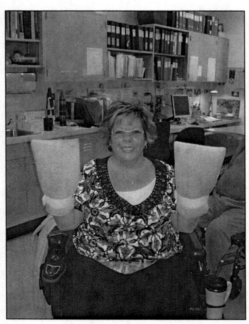

Wax on, wax off . . . we soaked my hands daily in hot wax, which helped my circulation return (I also bought a portable wax machine for home, which we used every night for many months).

Dear Suzan,

I want to thank you for sharing your wonderful spirit & outlook during your time here at Eagle Ridge. You have a rare gift of truly connecting with people & making people feel good. I know your deep faith has a lot to do with that. Lots of people have faith, but they keep it to themselves. You share & witness to others, & that is what makes your gift so rare & beautiful. You have an amazing story. I have no doubt this is part of God's greater plan for you & you were meant to be doing EXACTLY what you are doing. You have been on quite a journey, but you touch so many people in such a special way

– 2 –

as you are on this journey. I know you have touched me in a very profound way. I just want to say thank you. I have no doubt that God is looking down on you & your journey & thinking, "Well done, good and faithful servant."

I just wanted to thank you for the bright light and deep faith you have shared while you were here. You are definitely leaving a great gift behind with me as you continue on your journey. I wish you well, & I'll keep you in my prayers. God bless. Love,
Joanne

joko53@shaw.ca
keep in touch!

Joanne from Eagle Ridge Hospital gave me this card, which I treasure to this day. Thank you.

CHAPTER 35

Oh Happy Day! Buying Our First Home Together

This is was one of the best days of my life. After years of our family keeping our addresses in pencil in their address books because we moved around so often, we moved into our gorgeous waterfront condo in New Westminster, British Columbia—and now a pen could be used by all.

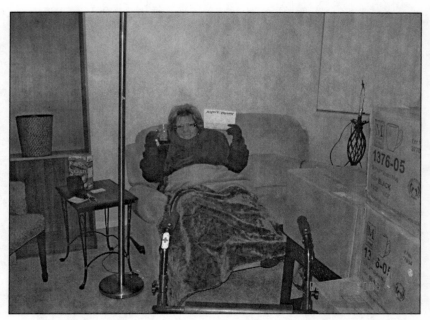

Moving-in night. We were exhausted, and the heat was not working fast enough for me. I look like a little Eskimo doll.

CHAPTER 36

Keeping My Deal with God

My neurologist, Dr. Chapman, asked if I would be willing to come and speak to the second-year medical students. The professor would speak about the technicalities of GBS, and then my neurologist would talk how the neuroanatomy and physiology applied to an actual patient: me. When we saw the questions they wanted me to answer, there were a few regarding the effect on my spouse. We felt it would be best for these "doctors to be" to hear that side of the story directly from John. So he came to the presentation. When we arrived, we had anticipated there would be around 40 persons in the theatre. However, more than 300 showed up. It was being live-video fed to University of Victoria and University of Northern British Columbia, so around 500 students were attending!

Talk about jumping right back onto the bicycle, but John and I did great and enjoyed hearing the feedback. There was this incredible moment that happened. At the end, after everyone clapped, gave us a standing ovation and thanked us, a gentleman named Nathan came up to me and said he'd had GBS when he was 10, had recovered well and had never met another GBS patient before. He was thrilled and shared with us that this is why he went into medicine—because his dream is to find a cure. Wow! Talk about a powerful moment.

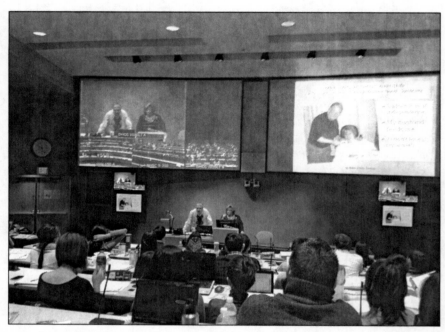

John and I speaking to the University of British Columbia second-year medical students (we have been asked back three times since then). Here is that deer-in-the-headlights look again.

CHAPTER 37

Giving Back—the Patient Becomes a Liaison

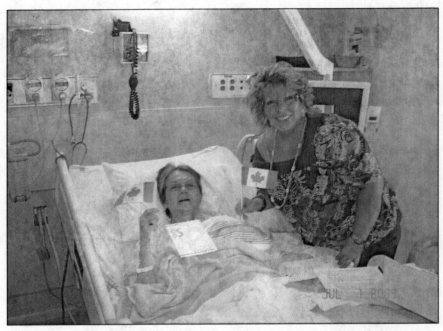

Working as a liaison with the Guillain-Barré Syndrome of Canada Foundation and visiting Beatrice in the hospital.

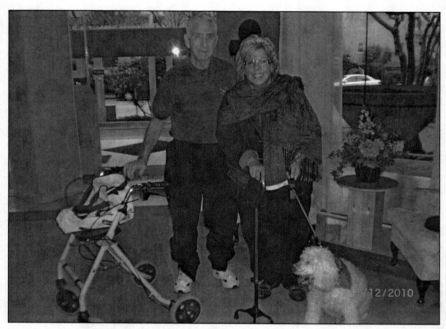

Here I am visiting Paul, with my companion, Kiki.

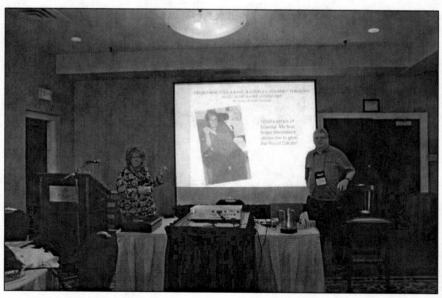

John and I were asked to give a presentation on our journey at our National GBS/CIDP Conference in Toronto, April 2011.

132

CHAPTER 38

Going Back

When I went back to G. F. Strong for my first post-discharge visit, I was really happy to see Walter. You see, one day, when I was still a patient, I was in a bit of a funk and just craving some kind of reassurance that I was going to be okay, Walter rolled in and introduced himself. He works with people who, like himself, suffer spinal cord trauma and was asked by our mutual friend, Randy, to pop in on me. He was a huge inspiration and explained life this way: "We are all loved by God and are all perfect little pieces that make up God's puzzle. Without any one of us, the puzzle can never be completed. God does not care if we have fingers or feet; he merely loves us just as we are." I thought this profound and began to cry. Not tears of sadness but tears of happiness, for I knew I was going to be okay. I will always hold a very warm spot in my heart for Walter, as he helped me through a terribly dark period.

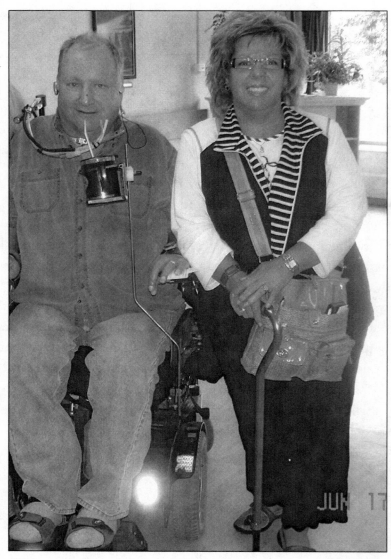

With very wise Walter. I don't think Walter will ever know what a profound role he played in my healing.

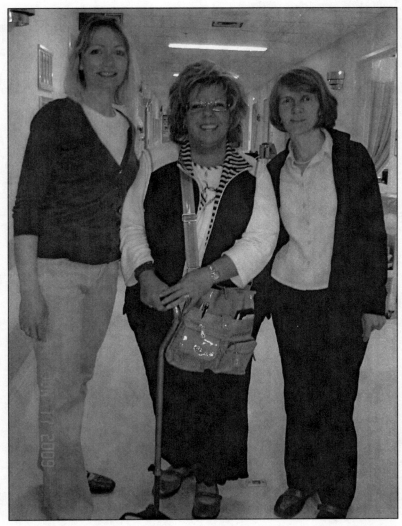

During this same visit, I was able to see Marian, my physiotherapist, and Isobel, my occupational therapist. It felt so fantastic to be "standing" next to them. I will always owe them a debt of gratitude because they never wavered in their support and encouragement.

"What do you do to stop the negative mental chatter? I will not listen to anyone more messed up than I am"

~Michael J. Fox~

CHAPTER 39

Thanks for the Encouragement and Support

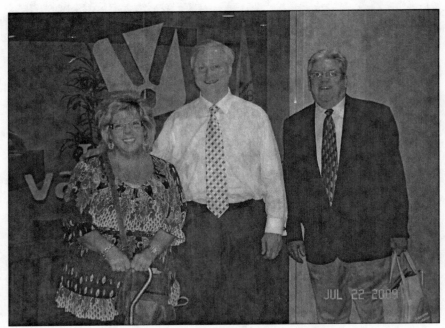

Our first stop in writing this book was visiting Rick, CEO Tourism Vancouver, who afforded us not only his time but his incredible vision and encouragement. Thanks, Rick.

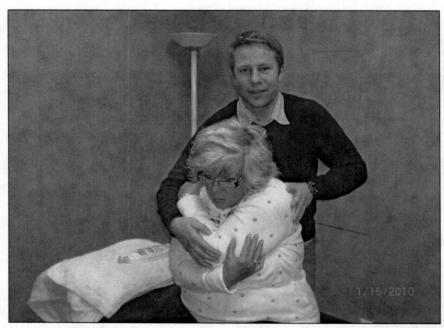

Trailside Physiotherapy: here is Kevin working his magic on my sore, aching body. I must say he sure looks like he is enjoying inflicting pain on me, doesn't he? My husband penned his nickname: "Prince of Pain."

CHAPTER 40

And Then They Came around the Corner

I had dreamed of this day for so long. Just a chance encounter, to bump into the various occupational and physiotherapists who formed my "team" and make them proud.

Several months after my discharge from G. F. Strong, I was at the Rehabilitation Expo in Vancouver, standing with my walker, at the booth where I was helping out and distributing GBS/CIDP information. Suddenly, the occupational therapy team from G. F. Strong Rehab Facility appeared. They took one look at me standing and their faces fell to the floor. Here I was, the "poster patient" for rehab and representing the actual reason they do what they do. When I walked over to them with my walker, there were serious tears shed. I was helping out at the CDIA (Canadian Disabled Individuals Association) booth and had come full circle. The last time these folks saw me was when I was discharged from their rehab facility, still heavily reliant on my power chair. And now I was standing at a tradeshow booth. Even now, when I think of that day, I still get goose bumps and misty eyed.

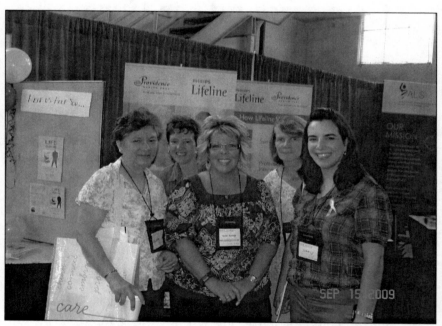

Happy group shot: reunited with the occupational therapists from G. F. Strong Rehabilitation Centre.

CHAPTER 41

Becoming an Advocate

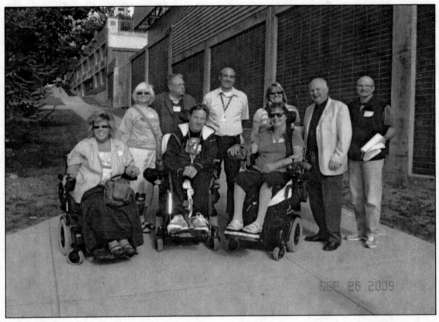

John and I took part in the "Wheelability" Assessment Project in New Westminster. Pictured from left in back row: Margie, John, John Stark, Gillie, Mayor Wayne Wright, and Greig. Front row: Suzan, Rick, Tanis

"When you can see obstacles for what they are, you never lose faith in the path it takes to get you where you want to go".

~Oprah Winfrey~

NEW WESTMINSTER

The Record

WEDNESDAY, SEPTEMBER 30, 2009

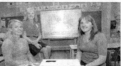

INSIDE FEATURE: Helping all students learn ▶P13

YOUR SOURCE FOR LOCAL SPORTS, NEWS, WEATHER AND ENTERTAINMENT! : WWW.ROYALCITYRECORD.COM

▶STAFF CUTS BLAMED

Parents complain after 'dirty Tuesday'

BY NIKI HOPE REPORTER
nhope@royalcityrecord.com

E.W. Howay Elementary School had a dirty day, and parents there are blaming it on staffing cuts.

A recent Tuesday was a particularly messy day at the school after a student entered a closed bathroom to vomit and ended up stepping in feces, which was then tracked through the school, Howay parent advisory council chair Andra Vowles explained.

Howay lost its day custodian this year. The school custodian's shift doesn't start until 3 p.m. so the bathroom was closed until a custodian arrived.

To offset a budget deficit, the district had to lay off a number of support staff, including two custodians. As a result, Howay lost its day custodian, who, up until last year, started at 10 a.m.

When the recent situation occurred at Howay, Vowles said the district was contacted and an urgent work order was issued, but no one turned up to clean the mess.

Also, because one bathroom was closed, there was a line-up of boys waiting to wash their hands after lunch in another, smaller bathroom. This concerns Vowles, who works in health care as a dietician, because of the threat of H1N1 and other seasonal viruses.

Every classroom in Howay has a sink, though Vowles said parents at the school would like to be able to use waterless hand cleaner. The alcohol-based cleaners have been banned from the school because of concerns around alcohol content and scent (a

▶School Page 30

'IT WAS A GREAT EYE-OPENER FOR EVERYBODY': MARIAM LARSON

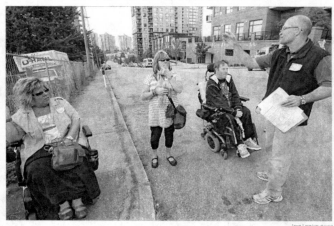

On a roll: From left, Suzan Jennings, Gillie Treeldge, Rick McArthur and team leader Greg Dedgsham, the city's streets supervisor, take part in a "wheelability" assessment near Douglas College, part of a city effort to help improve accessibility.

Test-driving city streets

BY THERESA McMANUS REPORTER
tmcmanus@royalcityrecord.com

A group of volunteers hit the streets on Saturday to check out the "wheelability" of the downtown.

The City of New Westminster is getting a better sense of the challenges faced by people with mobility aids through a pilot project that is assessing the wheelability of the uptown and downtown neighbourhoods. People with mobility aids such as wheelchairs and walkers were invited to participate.

Unless you have experienced it or are living with someone who has experienced it, you just don't think about it," said Mariam Larson, a gerontologist who is the project's facilitator. "It was a great eye-opener for everybody. Knowledge can lead to change."

On Sept. 12, participants did assessments of the uptown, and on Sept. 26 they took to the downtown. Small teams, each including a city staff representative, look to the streets to assess sidewalks, challenges crossing streets, areas that work well — or don't, and options to make access better.

It went really well," Larson said. "The metro were challenging because of the hills in the downtown. People were dedicated troopers."

The group of 27 participating in the Sept. 26 assessment included 12 mobility aid users. Those companions, the mayor and several city staff, and several members of the working group that's been overseeing the wheelability assessment project.

The two wheelability assessment days have included participation from more than 20 people with a range of mobility aids, including eight people with power chairs, five with scooters, five with manual wheelchairs, two with walkers and one with a cane. The men and women participating have ranged from 25 to over 80

▶Testing Page 4

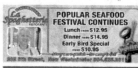
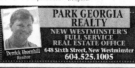
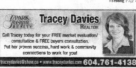
Article that appeared in the Royal City Record newspaper, September 30, 2009 about the "Wheelability" Assessment Project, written by Theresa McManus.

CHAPTER 42

Counting One's Blessings

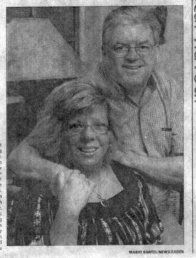

A reason to count one's blessings

Suzan Jennings walking tall dispite rare disorder

**Suzan and John Jennings'
Friday Night Picnic Recipe for chillin'**

INGREDIENTS

- 1 whole wheat baguette—Warmed and cut in thick slices, with butter, margarine or mayonnaise
- Sharp cheddar cheese—Cut into 1" pieces
- Danish blue cheese—Wedge with spreader
- Brie or camembert—Room temperature with spreader
- Tube of fine liver sausage—With spreader
- Garlic sausage ring—Cut into slices
- Assorted fresh veggies—Carrots, green and red pepper, celery, cherry tomatoes in bite-sized pieces—served with favourite dip or light ranch dressing
- Assorted fresh fruit—grapes, apples, orange or grapefruit—Cut in wedges
- Seasonal options:
  Summer-Homemade or store-bought potato salad
  Winter- Tomato or mushroom soup

Eighteen months ago, Suzan Jennings was, as she describes it, "fine, fab and forty-six." She was enjoying life with her husband, John, and their dog, Tiki. She had a busy job in the hospitality industry. She enjoyed going out to eat in restaurants. In March 2008, she noticed some tingling and numbness in the left side of her face. By the next day, it had spread to her left arm, then her left leg, making it difficult for her to walk. She went to her doctor, who dismissed her symptoms as stress. "Take a few days off and relax," she says he told her. A few days later she had no choice; she couldn't work anymore, she couldn't move at all. Her husband took her to the hospital, where she collapsed in the emergency room. Five spinal taps later, she was diagnosed with Guillain-Barre Syndrome, a rare autoimmune disorder of the nervous system that affects one or two people per 100,000. She spent six weeks at St. Paul's Hospital in Vancouver, getting treated with high-dose intravenous immunoglobulins. Her neurologist told her she'd likely never walk again. Jennings had other ideas. On May 7, 2008, she began three months of intensive physiotherapy at GF Strong Rehabilitation Facility. By August, she was well enough to go home. Following a regimen of physiotherapy, chiropractic treatments, massage therapy and aquacize, she's regained her ability to walk. "I really try to stay active and rest as much as possible," says Jennings. She's also giving back by volunteering as the Greater Vancouver liaison for the GBS Foundation to help others going through their own diagnosis. But the disease is so rare, her reach has extended to patients in the United States and even the Philippines. She's also working on a book about her journey to recovery. "To go from being healthy to completely paralyzed in a few days is very frightening," says Jennings. "Now my life is full of purpose in ways that I never could have dreamed of." Jennings says she doesn't feel at home in the kitchen—she lets her husband do most of the cooking. Or they eat out. But on Fridays, they like to relax, and count their blessings, by having a simple picnic in their living room.

MARIO BARTEL/NEWSLEADER

The New Westminster News Leader found out about our story and requested an interview. This is the story as it appeared October 29, 2009, written by Mario Bartel.

CHAPTER 43

Hubby Takes Me to Maui

John and I took our first holiday, post hospital, in Maui. We were blessed to be able to go for three wonderful weeks with our dear friends Don and Marilyn. We all agreed it was the best holiday ever. Great weather, great food and great friends.

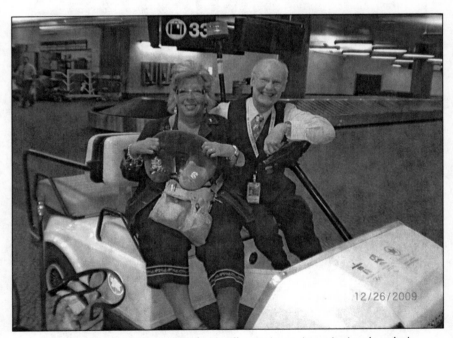

Here I am on our airline's "people mover" to assist me in navigating through the terminal to the departure gate.

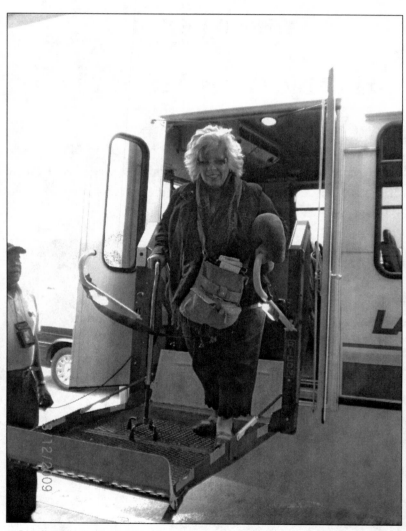

I really felt there should have a been a sign on me saying "wide load" because as I was coming down this transfer vehicle, it constantly beeped, just like a truck backing up!

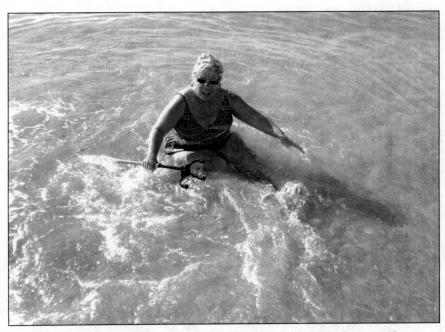

One minute I was wading into the shallow ocean beach, and then the next, a huge wave came over me and wham! I was down in the water and rolling around like a fish and squealing like a little girl, so much so that all these people came running to help me. I felt bad for everyone who thought I was drowning, but honestly, it was the best moment ever!

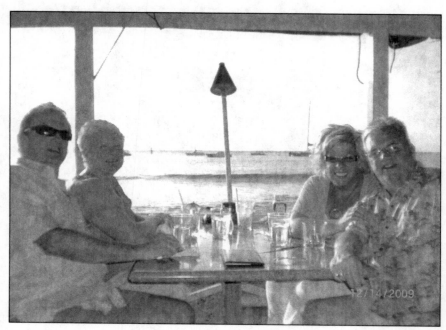

Enjoying a delicious oceanfront dinner with our travelling companions, Don and Marilyn, whom John went to high school with several decades previous. After this trip, Don suffered some health challenges, but we were able to return for another Maui vacation.

CHAPTER 44

The Vancouver 2010 Olympics

The Olympics came to town and the torch passed right by our home. I was able to attend an Olympic luncheon and even held the torch and John drove VIPs around the Olympic venues.

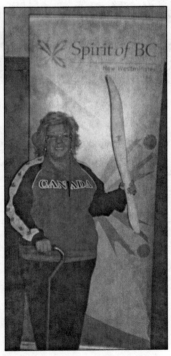

I attended an Olympic luncheon and was thrilled to have an opportunity to hold the torch. I just love this photo because even though I was not a world-class athlete, I felt like a winner who had won a race!

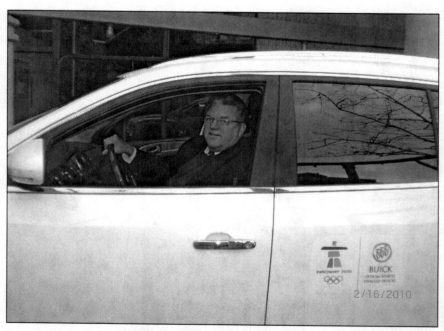

John drove VIPs around the various Olympic sites. He looks so handsome in his vehicle.

CHAPTER 45

And Then There Was Lady

After losing Kiki in August 2010, we were not sure if we would ever have another "forever friend" because he was such a huge part of my recovery and a great companion to us both. Several months later, John looked at me and said, "We need to go find a new friend." I canvassed all the dog rescue sites looking for just the one, and we found her at our local BCSPCA. We do not know everything she went through but suffice to say, we are all survivors, and Lady is the gift that just keeps on giving.

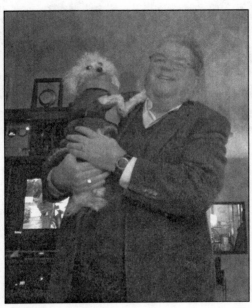

Daddy and his little girl.

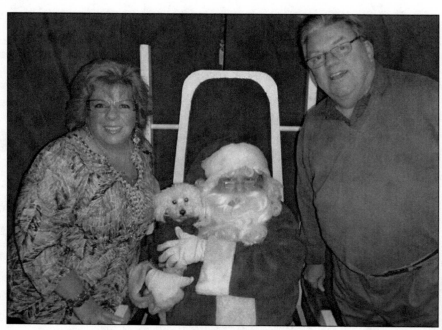

Santa really outdid himself with our gift—Lady.

CHAPTER 46

Knee Replacement Surgery

When I came out of paralysis and began walking in rehab, I experienced such pain that I was sent for an MRI. What the film showed was that I had absolutely no tissue or cartilage in my left knee and only a small amount left in my right knee. Knee replacement surgery was urgent to continue on my path of recovery. Having surgery and being in the hospital posed several concerns for me, as one of the by-products of Guillain-Barré syndrome is a compromised immune system. The surgery was a success, I guess, but I suffered a number of setbacks such as inadequate healing, incision infection and medication reactions to morphine and oxycodone.

I ended up checking out of the hospital two days early because I was squeezed into a double room with two other patients with C. Difficile bacterium infection and were highly contagious. It seemed I was the only one concerned about this, and the nurses simply told me not to touch anything!

Once home, John had many laughs because I suffered through many hallucinations. For example, we were sitting in the living room watching TV, and I was apparently having a perfectly good conversation with no one. John said he felt left out so he was contributing to the conversation wherever he could, but he said it was hard getting a word in! Another time I was walking down the hall going to the washroom and I said excuse me to no one there!

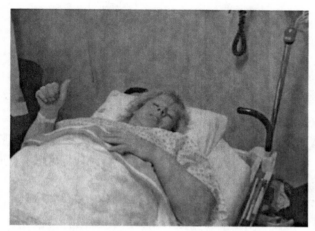

A few minutes before the drugs kicked in. We are off like a herd of turtles.

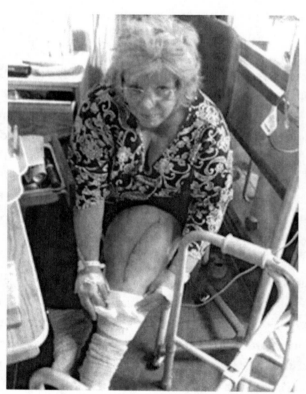

I jokingly asked my surgeon if he had fallen asleep or was intoxicated because the incision starts straight and then veers off course.

CHAPTER 47

Isolation

funny thing happened on the road to recovery. It was like I went from being voted "most popular" while in the hospital to being confined to isolation when I went home. While in the hospital, the nurses often commented on how they had never seen so many people visit one patient before and that I must have had a very large family. The ironic fact here is that both John and I lost our parents at a young age, and I only have one brother and sister-in-law, and an aunt and cousins who all live in Victoria. Other than that, it was our extended "family of friends" who championed my recovery.

Dealing with my isolation is something I am still working on to this day. I find myself saying I haven't heard from this person or that person for a very long time, and more often than not, I will pick up the phone and call them. My point is, if I didn't do this, I would not hear from them. I have asked a few friends why they don't call, and they have said it's because they didn't want to bother us!

I finally figured out that this occurred and it was nobody's fault. Oprah wrote, "Anything can be a miracle, a blessing, an opportunity if you choose to see it that way. When you can see obstacles for what they are, you never lose faith in the path it takes to get you where you want to go."

When I was first admitted to the hospital, it took everyone by surprise and I was "top of mind." What I must remember is that everyone was there for us when we needed them most, and now that I am getting better and out of hospital, they have returned to their own lives.

I read this saying somewhere, and it seemed apropos: "When others want you to do well, you come out of your isolation."

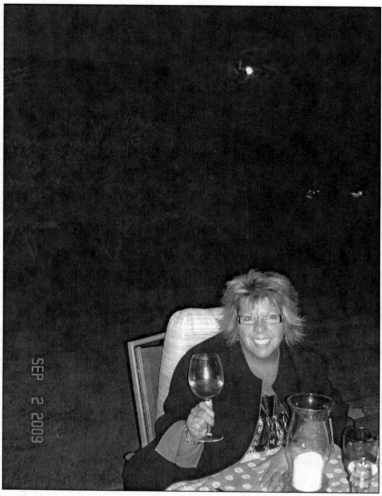

All by myself . . .

EPILOGUE

Since that day—March 31, 2008—I have had many highs and lows. I had a wonderful life, and then all of a sudden my whole life changed. Just like that. I never had a chance to catch my breath.

I sobbed the day I was admitted and finally brought to my room and the intake nurse said to me, "I hope you said good-bye to your husband because he won't be back!" I sobbed the day I had a brief sensation in my right hand and then it disappeared. I sobbed the day I was almost denied admittance to the rehabilitation centre. I sobbed the day my care team told me it was unlikely I would ever walk again or have use of my hands. I sobbed many days after that as well.

God answered me that fateful day by providing me with more strength to forge ahead. Today I am an active liaison for the Guillain-Barré Foundation of Canada, and in fact, April 2011, we were asked to give a presentation about our journey at the national conference in Toronto.

With my level of recovery, John was able to re-enter the workplace with confidence that I could be left on my own. This has been important to him, and he is now truly finding his own "confident" self. I am able to volunteer on a flexible basis, to help others and become a champion to persons with disabilities. I also am involved in our local community's accessibility improvement projects and transportation system.

The recovery period in GBS can vary from weeks to years, depending on the severity of the illness. Although I have recovered remarkably well, I have many leftover residual symptoms, such as tingling mixed with sharp jolts of pain, which feel like I am being electrocuted in my hands, feet, neck and shoulders and down my spine. I now have restless leg syndrome, and my eyesight has become impaired by blurry double vision. My balance did not return, and I require the use of a walking aid for short outings and a wheelchair for long outings. A high level of pain has continued to plague me, which requires an ever-changing cocktail of medications. There continue to be many days where I possess such a high level of fatigue it limits my ability to perform regular, everyday tasks. I am now "permanently disabled" and have reached my plateau, whereby, although I continue with my physical therapy and fitness activities, I have not and probably will not see much further improvement.

In May 2011 we went back to my hometown, Ottawa, Ontario, and visited some friends and got reacquainted with many of my family that I have not seen since my father's passing in June 2003 or even longer. It was really wonderful to feel loved and missed by them.

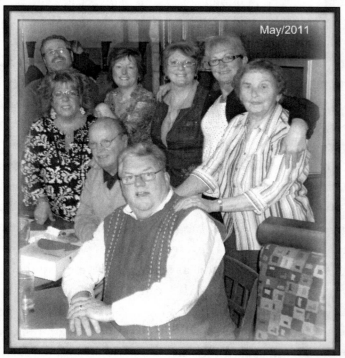

Family dinner with my uncle Bobby, aunt Terry and cousins Linda, Joanne, Carolle and Alain.

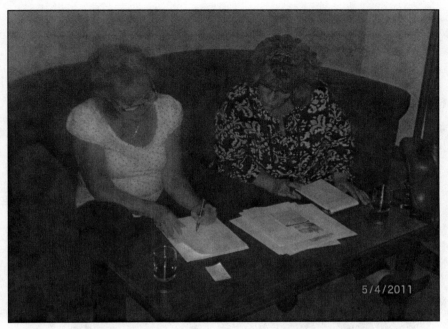

This is one of my favourite moments to date: my cousin Carolle was helping us edit our first draft, and for the first time, I felt that writing our book could become a reality.

Before John and I left Ottawa, we visited Notre Dame Cemetery, where my mom and dad are buried. I felt extremely emotional because it was the first time I had seen both their names on the headstone, as my mom passed away March 1987 and my father June 2003. May you both rest in peace.

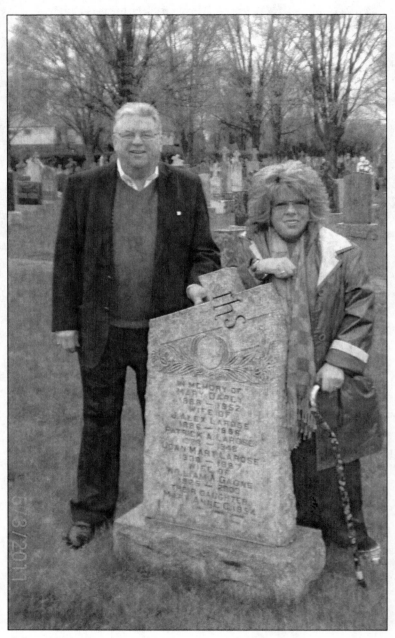

John and I visit the cemetery where my parents are buried.

During those dark days in the hospital, I would stare at the clock, watch the hands move, listen to it go tick, tick, tick and would wonder how much time had elapsed. Wondering what would happen to me if I fell asleep. What would happen to me when I woke up? Would I wake up? Would I be worse? What I have learned to do is focus on what I can do and not what I used to be able to do. I set targets and goals and then try to keep them. Yes, I have had many ups and downs, but that target moves me on and pushes me harder than I ever thought possible; like writing this book. Some days I did not have hands to write, and other days I did not have eyes to see, but I never—okay, almost never—lost my dream of seeing our journey put on paper. If at the end of the day one person is inspired or has just simply enjoyed what we wrote or has realized he or she wasn't living a "best, purpose-driven life," then it was not all in vain.

Like losing a loved one, I have had to mourn the "old" me and my "old" life. The old me that I had known for 46 years had a career, drove a car and was fearless. The quick paralysis and helpless state of dependence on others for the most basic human needs left me feeling as if I had lost my dignity and worried I would never find it again. I felt lost and found it hard to find my way back. It was excruciating to watch my husband watch me deteriorate and then struggle through the slow recovery process. When I was released from G. F. Strong for the recovery phase, my husband was overwhelmed to find himself in complete charge of a patient who could not walk and who required large amounts of medications at regular intervals, all the while struggling with the uncertainty of this strange illness that attacks often in minutes or hours and sometimes in days or weeks. I guess we have both had to mourn our old life and our old relationship.

Steve Jobs passed away at the age of 56, and I read a quote from him that said, "If you live each day as if it was your last, someday you'll most certainly be right." How I have persevered and continued to thrive is because of my faith in God and the belief that I am stronger than I thought I was, that I am fine now and that I will be fine in the future.

I had a handle on life; then the handle broke, but now the handle has been repaired through the power of faith.

Throughout our journey, we have found out what is important in life, which is our new focus. Relationships come in different sizes and colours, and we have a long way to go but are making a conscious decision to work at it because it is not going to fix itself. We put a lot of pressure on having relationships that are perfect, and when you have been through a sudden change in life, there is no such thing as perfect.

A professor from the University of British Columbia that we know from our inspirational talks to the medical students recommended us to Percy, a reporter from the CNN network. After we discussed our story with Percy, he decided there was a story there and that he would like to film it. We were just so excited that he had chosen to film our journey, and then we started the task of putting all the pieces together required, like our story outline and corresponding photos.

As my 50th birthday was fast approaching, a party celebrating "Suzan turns 50 against all odds" would be fantastic. Not only would he film my actual party, he would interview various friends and family for the documentary/drama. John had a delicious cake made up, which said, "Happy Birthday, Suzan . . . you have survived and now you have arrived at your big 50! All our love." It was fabulous, and more than 30 of our closest family and friends were there to celebrate with us. Additionally we returned to G. F. Strong to film a re-enactment portion and our individual on-air segments.

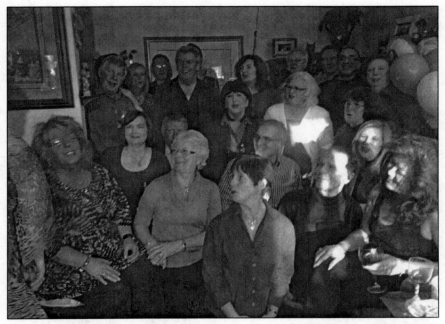

We had more than 30 friends at our home to celebrate my 50th and be there for the filming.

We felt truly blessed that our story could very well be featured on CNN, and our dream is to provide hope and inspiration to anyone out there who may be in a crisis situation right now. As of this date of writing, we have not heard when it will air, but we can't wait.

This past February 2012, I said to John one day, "Why don't you retire and enjoy life?"

John thought this an intriguing proposition, and this propelled us into the most exciting and frustrating five months of our lives.

Once we listed our home for sale, our realtor and friends all thought our house would sell within a short period. This did not happen. Nineteen open houses and 17 separate showings later, we finally had a solid offer, but only after significantly dropping our price.

At this point, we had to say, *so what was our objective anyway?* We knew, hands down, our objective was to move into an area that could provide a "forever" peace of quiet and safe minds, and we were able to achieve that by purchasing our wonderful patio home in the Oceanside community of Parksville, on Vancouver Island. We both have agreed this was the most taxing move we had ever experienced, because for the first time, we were all alone to unpack and arrange our home. Although this prospect was and still is daunting at times, it has been the most rewarding because we have carved out a lovely piece of heaven that the three of us are blessed to have.

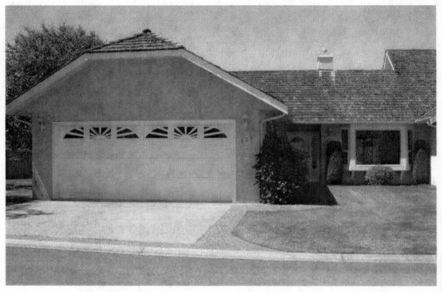

When we were looking for our "forever home," we both were adamant in our wants and needs. I absolutely wanted single-level living, and John wanted a double-sized attached garage. We both got what we wished for and so much more.

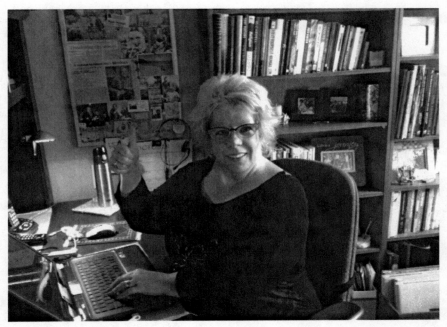

Here I am creating this "work of art" in our writing room! We had been working on this manuscript for more than three years and at times thought it would never finish, but we never lost faith.

"If you really believe life is a journey, then you recognize that not all journeys follow straight roads. You can count on the curves, bumps, detours, uphill climbs and even the downhill slides".

~Oprah Winfrey~

"Making a difference . . . one step at a time" has become my personal mantra. This is our story, and we believe it is never too late to find meaning in one's life. Thank you for taking this journey with us.

~Suzan & John~

GUILLAIN-BARRÉ
SYNDROME FACT SHEET

What is Guillain-Barré Syndrome? Guillain-Barré syndrome (GBS) is rare disorder in which the body's immune system attacks part of the peripheral nervous system. The first symptoms of this disorder include varying degrees of weakness or tingling sensations in the legs. In many instances, the weakness and abnormal sensations spread to the arms and upper body. These symptoms can increase in intensity until the muscles cannot be used at all and the patient is almost totally paralyzed. In these cases, the disorder is life-threatening and is considered a medical emergency. The patient is often put on a ventilator to assist with breathing. Most patients, however, recover from even the most severe cases of Guillain-Barré syndrome, although some continue to have some degree of weakness.

Guillain-Barré syndrome is rare. It usually occurs a few days or weeks after the patient has had symptoms of a respiratory or gastrointestinal viral infection. Occasionally, surgery will trigger the syndrome. In rare instances, vaccinations may increase the risk of GBS. The disorder can develop over the course of hours or days, or it may take up to three to four weeks. No one yet knows why Guillain-Barré strikes some people and not others or what sets the disease in motion.

What scientists do know is that the body's immune system begins to attack the body itself, causing what is known as an autoimmune disease. Guillain-Barré is called a syndrome rather than a disease because it is not clear that a specific disease-causing agent is involved. Reflexes such as knee jerks are usually lost. Because the signals travelling along the nerve are slower, a nerve conduction velocity (NCV) test can give doctor clues to aid the diagnosis. The cerebrospinal fluid that bathes the spinal cord and brain contains more protein than usual, so a physician may decide to perform a spinal tap. Though rare, GBS is the most common cause of rapidly acquired paralysis and affects 1 person per 100,000. The disorder came to public attention briefly when it struck a number of people who received the 1976 swine flu vaccine and continues to claim thousands of new victims each year, striking any person, at any age, regardless of gender or ethnic background, making GBS difficult to predict or study.

Is there any treatment? There is no known cure for Guillain-Barré syndrome, but therapies can lessen the severity of the illness and accelerate the recovery in most patients. There are also a number of ways to treat the complications of the disease. Currently, plasmapheresis (also known as plasma exchange) and high-dose IVIG immunoglobulin therapy are used. Plasmapheresis seems to reduce the severity and duration of the Guillain-Barré episode. In high-dose IVIG immunoglobulin therapy, doctors give intravenous injections of the proteins that in small quantities, the immune system uses naturally to attack invading organism. Investigators have found that giving high doses of these immunoglobulins, derived from a pool of thousands of normal donors, to Guillain-Barré patients can lessen the immune attack on the nervous system. The most critical part of the treatment for this syndrome consists of keeping the patient's body functioning during recovery of the nervous system. This can sometimes require placing the patient on a ventilator, a heart monitor or other machines that assist body function.

What is the prognosis? Guillain-Barré syndrome can be a devastating disorder because of its sudden and unexpected onset. Most people reach the stage of greatest weakness within the first two weeks after symptoms appear, and by the third week of the illness 90 percent of all patients are at their weakest. The recovery period may be as little as a few weeks or as long as a few years. About 30 percent of those with Guillain-Barré still have a residual weakness after three years. About 3 percent may suffer a relapse of muscle weakness and tingling sensations many years after the initial attack.

What research is being done? Scientists are concentrating on finding new treatments and refining existing ones. Scientists are also looking at the workings of the immune system to find which cells are responsible for beginning and carrying out the attack on the nervous system. The fact that so many cases of Guillain-Barré begin after a viral or bacterial infection suggests that certain characteristics of some viruses and bacteria may activate the immune system inappropriately. Investigators are searching for those characteristics. Neurological scientists, immunologists, virologists, and pharmacologists are all working collaboratively to learn how to prevent this disorder and to make better therapies available when it strikes.

Reprinted From:
NINDS National Institute of Neurological Disorders and Strokes; NIH Neurological Institute: www.ninds.nih.gov

CPSIA information can be obtained at www.ICGtesting.com
Printed in the USA
LVOW11s2312270214

375450LV00002B/21/P